FUNDAMENTALS OF Uroradiology

Michael R. Williamson, M.D.
Chief Diagnostic Ultrasound
University of New Mexico
School of Medicine
Albuquerque, New Mexico

Anthony Y. Smith, M.D.
Associate Professor
Surgery/Urology/Transplant
University of New Mexico
Albuquerque, New Mexico

W.B. SAUNDERS COMPANY
A Division of Harcourt Brace and Company
Philadelphia London Sydney Toronto

W.B. SAUNDERS COMPANY

A Division of Harcourt Brace & Company

The Curtis Center
Independence Square West
Philadelphia, Pennsylvania 19106

Library of Congress Cataloging-in-Publication Data

Williamson, Michael R.
Fundamentals of uroradiology / Michael R. Williamson, Anthony Y. Smith—1st ed.
p. cm.
ISBN 0-7216-5399-5
1. Urinary organs—Radiography. I. Smith, Anthony Y.
[DNLM: 1. Urography—methods. WJ 141 W7311f2000]
RC874.W54 2000
616.6′0754—dc21

99-044545

FUNDAMENTALS OF URORADIOLOGY ISBN 0-7216-5399-5

Printed in the United States of America

Last digit is the print number: 9 8 7 6 5 4 3 2 1

To my family

M. R. W.

For Sheila, Cameron, Sheldon

A. Y. S.

Preface

This book is intended to provide a core text for those who are just beginning their training in radiology or urology. The length is such that it can be read in a matter of hours. The illustrations have been chosen to demonstrate commonly encountered problems in uroradiology. This book may also be valuable for those who desire a quick review of the subject. Finally, family practitioners and emergency physicians may utilize it as a quick reference. This book is not intended to be a comprehensive text on the subject. Thanks are in order to Floyd Willard, Maureen Drexel, Joseph Tofoya, Gabriela Miranda, and Bernadette Pierce. Thanks are due Sara Langwell for her wonderful illustrations. This book was possible only with the support of Fred Mettler and Tom Borden.

Contents

Chapter

1

Normal Upper Tract

INTRODUCTION

Contrast agents are divided into ionic and nonionic types. Ionic agents have been in use for many years and are inexpensive but have an incidence of complications several times greater than that of nonionic agents. A downward trend in the price of the nonionic agents has resulted in a tendency to use them more often.

NORMAL UPPER TRACT

Contrast Agents

An intravenous urogram (IVU) is performed using contrast material with iodine as its essential agent (Table 1–1). A bolus of iodinated contrast material is administered intravenously. The peak plasma level is achieved immediately after injection. As the contrast material diffuses into the tissues and is excreted, the plasma level declines. Key factors determining the quality of the exam are the amount of iodine injected, the rate of injection, and the distention of the pelvicalyceal system. Distention of the pelvicalyceal system can be achieved by a compression band placed at the iliac crest. Excretion of contrast material depends on glomerular filtration alone. This is true for both high- and low-osmolality forms of contrast.

High-osmolality contrast agents cause an osmotic diuresis. These contrast agents generally consist of iodine bound to a benzene ring, which is in turn bound to a salt such as meglumine or sodium. Sodium salts produce a higher concentration of contrast material in the urine because the sodium will be partially reabsorbed in the tubules, causing less diuresis. Reabsorption in the tubules causes water reabsorption and a higher concentration of the contrast agent in the urine. Dehydration produces more nephrotoxicity, probably because of increased concentration of contrast material in the distal tubule.

Low-osmolality contrast agents concentrate in the urine but may have the undesirable side effect of obscuring collecting system abnormalities. In addition, less diuresis produces less distention.

Adults with normal renal function need 25 to 30 g of iodine or about 300 mg/kg body weight to visualize the kidney and collecting system. Practically, this corresponds to about 1 mL/kg for most of the common contrast agents. More contrast material may be neces-

TABLE 1–1. **Commonly Used Contrast Material for Excretory Urography and Computed Tomography**

Generic Name	Trade Name	Sodium Content (mEq/mL)	Iodine Content (mg/mL)	Osmolality (mOsm/kg H_2O)
Ionic Monomers				
Sodium diatrizoate	Hypaque 50	0.8	300	1515
Meglumine and sodium diatrizoate	Renografin 60	0.16	292	1420
Sodium iothalamate	Conray 400	1.05	400	2300
Meglumine iothalamate	Conray		282	1400
Nonionic Monomers				
Iopamidol	Isovue 300		300	616
Iohexol	Omnipaque		300	709
Ioversol	Optiray		320	702
Iopromide	Ultravist		300	620
Ioxilan	Oxilan		300	585
Ionic Dimer				
Meglumine and sodium ioxaglate	Hexabrix	0.15	320	600

Source: Modified from Davidson A, Hartman D, Radiology of the Kidney and Urinary Tract. WB Saunders, Philadelphia, PA, 1994. Reprinted with permission.

sary for patients with obesity or large amounts of stool in the bowel. An upper limit for contrast administration is 1 mL/lb body weight. In children, weight and age are both important determinants of dose (Table 1–2).

Some special considerations exist for contrast administration. A low-osmolality contrast agent is more desirable in children to prevent rapid volume expansion and resultant cardiac complications. Rapid or bolus injection of contrast material gives a better plasma level of iodine and a better-quality study. If there is an increased risk of cardiotoxicity, slower infusion over 2 or 3 minutes may reduce this risk. Patients who have heart disease have more diffusion into the extracellular fluid spaces. Older patients have a lower glomerular filtration rate, possibly because of reduced nephron mass. Opacification of the kidneys and collecting system will be reduced unless higher doses of contrast material are used.

TABLE 1–2. **Recommended Doses of Contrast Material for Pediatric Patients**

Weight (kg)	Dose
Up to 5.5	4.0 mL/kg
5.5 to 11.5	25 mL
11.5 to 23	2.0 mL/kg
23 to 46	50 mL
More than 46	1.0 mL/kg

Source: Davidson A, Hartman D, Radiology of the Kidney and Urinary Tract. WB Saunders, Philadelphia, PA, 1994. Reprinted with permission.

Adverse reactions may include systemic reactions that are minor or major. Minor reactions include hot flushes, nausea and vomiting, or urticaria. These usually resolve spontaneously or are easily treated by antihistamines. Major complications include bronchospasm, hypotension, laryngeal edema, cardiac arrest, and cardiopulmonary collapse. The overall incidence of contrast reactions is estimated at 13 percent with high-osmolality agents and 3 percent with low-osmolality agents. Organ-specific reactions can include nephrotoxicity with azotemia, myocardial ischemia, cardiac arrhythmia, ventricular tachycardia and fibrillation, and myocardial infarction. Major reactions are estimated to occur in 1 in 200 to 1 in 2000 patients with high-osmality contrast agents and in 1 in 640 to 1 in 2500 patients with low-osmolality agents. Fatal reactions are estimated to occur for 1 in 40,000 to 1 in 169,000 patients with high-osmolality agents and approximately 1 in 169,000 with low-osmolality agents.

Patients with certain risk factors have a

higher incidence of reactions. Any history of allergies such as hay fever, asthma, or hives increases the risk. Asthma is associated with an eightfold increased risk. A prior reaction to contrast material is associated with an 11-fold increased risk. Pretreatment reduces the risk of using high-osmolality agents. Our pretreatment regimen in adults consists of 50 mg of prednisone at 13, 7, and 1 hour before the exam, plus 50 mg of diphenhydramine 1 hour before the exam.

Renal toxicity may occur as acute tubular necrosis in association with low-flow states such as congestive heart failure or, more often, in patients with diabetes mellitus and prior renal impairment. Diabetics without prior renal impairment do not have associated renal toxicity. The renal toxicity manifests as an increase in creatinine and a decrease in creatinine clearance. These values may not return to baseline. Renal toxicity can also occur due to obstruction of the tubular lumen. This is seen in patients with multiple myeloma or with high uric acid levels and can be avoided by prior hydration. Low-osmolality contrast agents do not reduce the nephrotoxicity. A lower dose of iodine is the best means to minimize nephrotoxicity risk.

A routine intravenous urogram at our medical center consists of an immediate film of the kidneys taken at 2 minutes and a second film of the kidneys, ureters, and bladder taken at 5 minutes. We usually do three tomographic cuts through the kidneys at approximately 5 minutes after the injection of contrast. If no obstruction is seen, ureteral compression is applied and a film of the abdomen and pelvis is taken at 10 minutes to include the kidney, ureters, and bladder. If this film is satisfactory, compression is released. If the ureters or portions of the kidneys are not adequately visualized, right posterior and left posterior oblique images are obtained. The last film consists of an upright postvoid film of the pelvis.

Normal Intravenous Urogram

Renal size depends partially on patient size but is also influenced by patient age. Renal size is also influenced by the renal orientation in the body because the kidney is only measured in one plane. If the kidney is slightly rotated, it can appear foreshortened. When measured on an intravenous urogram, the right kidney should be no more than 1.5 cm longer than the left kidney. Since the left kidney is usually the larger kidney, it should be no more than 2 cm larger than the right. Kidneys should be about 3½ vertebral bodies in length. We use an upper limit of 14 cm for renal length and a lower limit of 9 cm. Subjective adjustments in the limits may be made for body size—e.g., little people have little kidneys (Fig. 1–1).

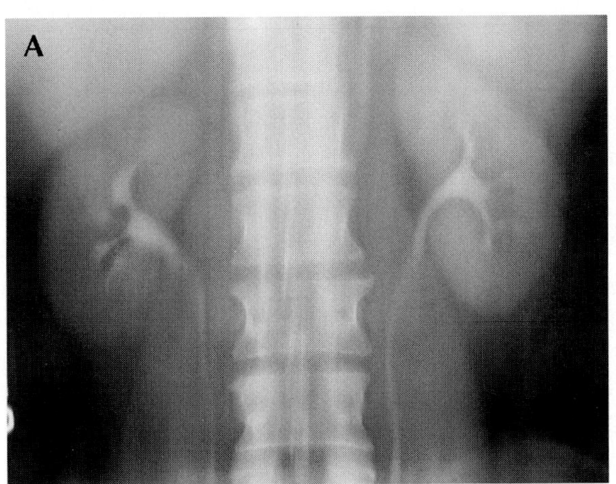

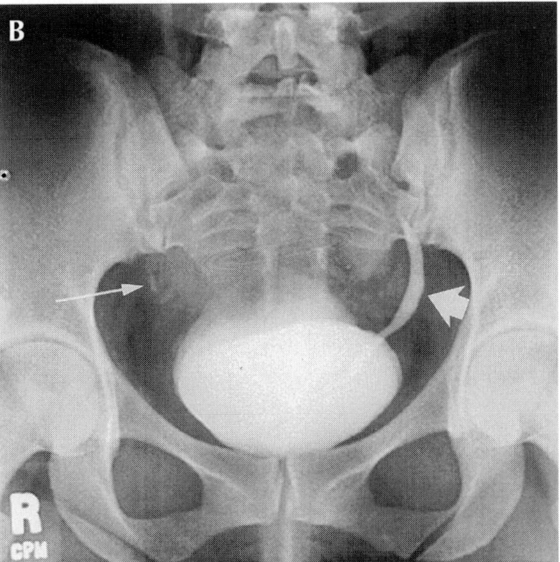

Figure 1–1. A. A normal 5-minute tomogram. **B.** A normal intravenous urogram. Film of a pelvis at 15 minutes shows the bladder filled with contrast material. The distal left ureter is well seen (large arrow), but only a small part of the right ureter is seen.

Generally, the contour of the kidneys is smooth. One normal variation is known as a dromedary hump. This a bulge on the lateral border of the left kidney and is felt to be a normal variant, probably secondary to compression of the developing kidney by the adjacent spleen (Fig. 1–2). Usually the kidney has a smooth contour, but at times there may be small, smooth, regular indentations or lobulations on the margin of the kidney. These are referred to as fetal lobulations and are felt to be a result of incomplete fusion of the embryologic fetal renal lobules. Fetal lobulations are to be distinguished from renal cortical scars and infarctions, which tend to be random and irregular. A prominent indentation along the superior aspect of the kidney is sometimes called a junctional defect or a sulcus interpartialis defect (Fig. 1–3).

On the average, approximately 13 to 14 calyces will be identified in a kidney, although the normal range is quite wide. Calyces are frequently grouped into three, with one group draining the upper pole, a second group draining the lower pole, and third group draining the midportion of the kidney. Calyces should have sharp margins. A rule of thumb is that the forniceal angles should be so sharp that you can "pick your fingernails" with them. Occasionally a blush of contrast material in the papilla adjacent to the calyx may be seen. This is highly concentrated iodine in distal collecting tubules and is a normal finding. Another normal calyceal variant is compression of the renal pelvis and calyces by fat. Fat will appear relatively lucent on a plain film and may appear echogenic on an ultrasound. This finding is more common in older patients and is referred to as renal sinus lipomatosis (Fig. 1–4).

The ureters may not be visualized in their entirety. However, portions of both ureters should be visualized on some of the films. One goal of a good intravenous urogram is to visualize all portions of both ureters, but this is not always technically possible. A ureter that is seen in its entirety on any one film may indicate pathology and is sometimes referred to as a "standing column" of contrast (Fig. 1–5). A standing col-

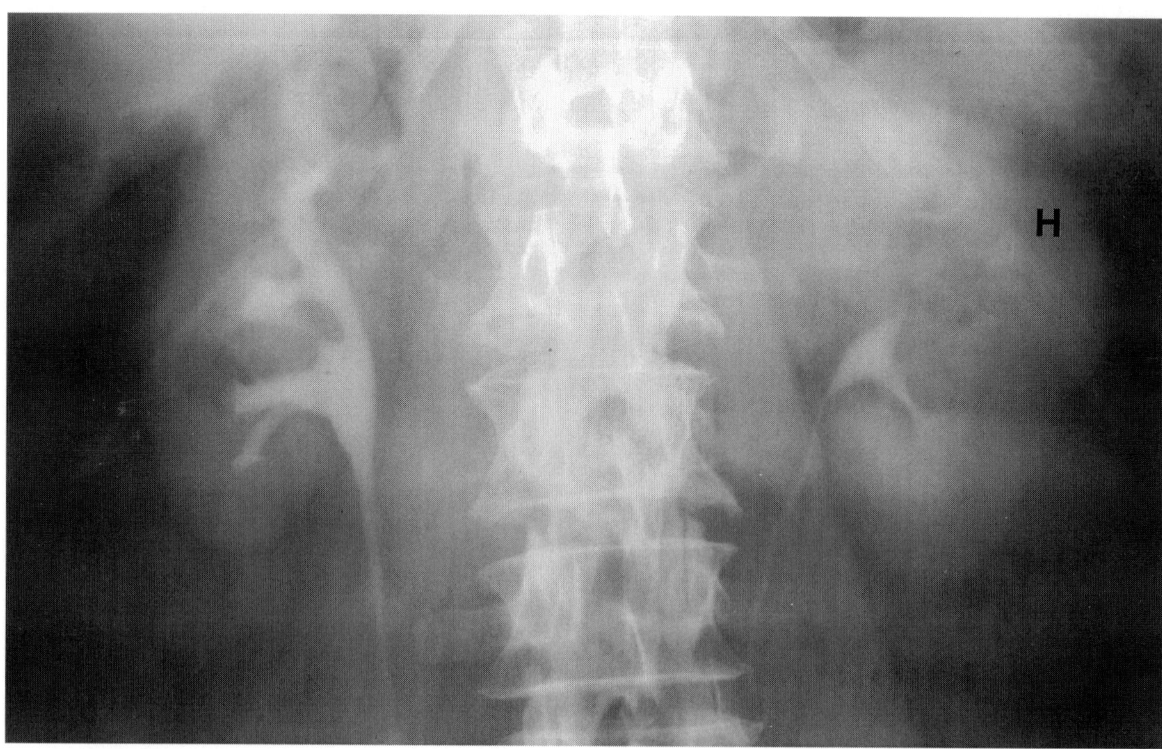

Figure 1–2. An intravenous urogram (IVU) showing a dromedary hump (H). This forms as a result of pressure from the adjacent spleen.

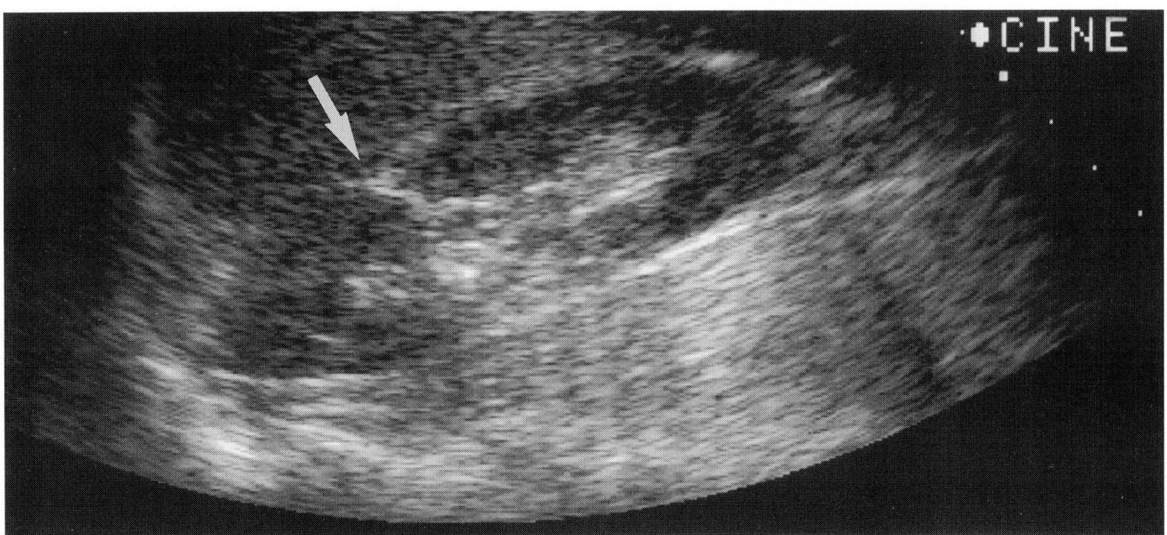

Figure 1–3. This longitudinal ultrasound image of the right kidney shows an indentation (arrow) at the junction between the upper third and the lower two-thirds of the kidney. This is a remnant of the way in which the kidney forms embryologically.

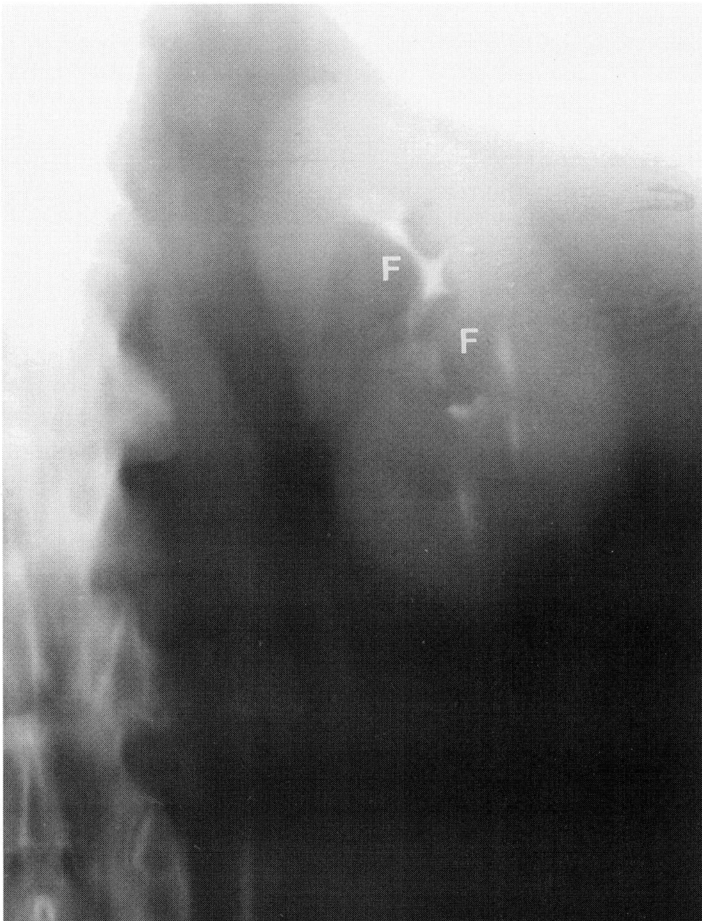

Figure 1–4. Renal sinus lipomatosis. The tomogram shows low-density material in the central portion of the left kidney. This is fat (F).

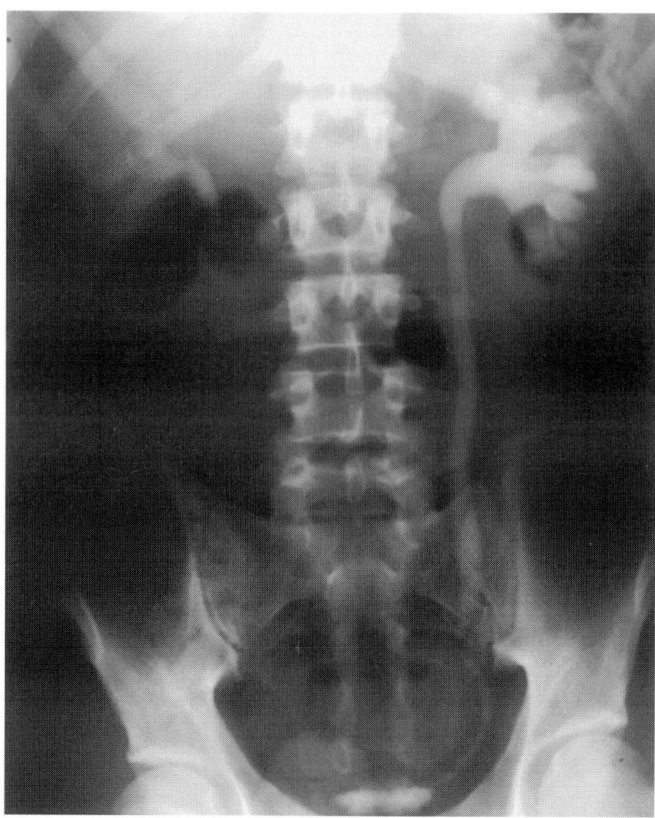

Figure 1–5. An intravenous urogram, 10-minute film. The left kidney has a standing column of contrast. This indicates obstruction even though no stone is seen.

umn of contrast may indicate either obstruction or the recent passage of a stone.

The normal bladder should have an elliptical to spherical shape. Irregularities in the shape of the bladder suggest either an extrinsic mass compressing the bladder or an intrinsic mass arising from the bladder wall. Oblique films may be helpful. Postvoid radiographs should show only a small amount of contrast remaining in the bladder.

Computed Tomography

Computed tomography (CT) provides a more thorough evaluation of the kidneys (Fig. 1–6). To image the kidneys for renal masses, CT scans are obtained both before and after contrast with thin cuts through the kidneys. We obtain 8-mm cuts of the kidneys before contrast. A bolus of 100 mL of IV contrast is given, and, after a 45-second delay, a second set of 5-mm cuts is performed. The precontrast images allow identification of stones and calcified structures. Stones that are not radiopaque on a standard kidney, ureter, and bladder x ray (KUB) should be easily seen on a CT scan because of its superior contrast resolution. Oral contrast may be given to opacify the bowel before a CT scan of the kidneys because loops of bowel cause confusion when evaluating renal masses and masses around the kidney. If the IV contrast is administered as a bolus, both arteries and veins may frequently be identified. With 5-mm cuts, the study should be sufficient to rule out renal vein thrombosis.

Hydronephrosis of the kidneys may be difficult to appreciate on a renal CT because of problems in determining whether a calyx is truly distended. Also, the renal pelvis may look dilated when it is simply extrarenal. It is important to examine the ureters from the kidney to the bladder to look for ureterectasis.

Computed tomography is being widely utilized to look for obstructing stones in patients with flank pain. The spiral CT technique is used to acquire data from about T11 (top of kidneys) through the

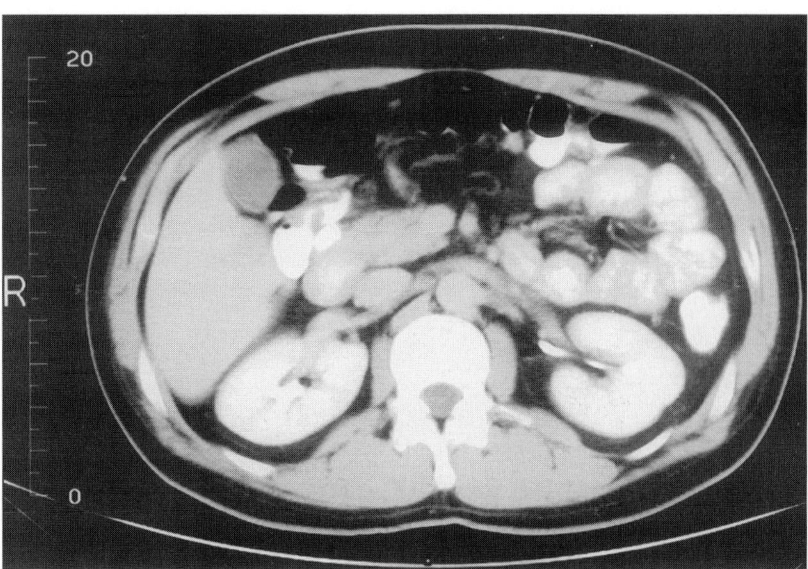

Figure 1–6. This postcontrast CT image shows normal kidneys.

pubic symphysis. Five-millimeter-thick images are then reconstructed. Signs of stone disease include identification of the stone, hydronephrosis, inflammatory "stranding" around the kidney, and a thick-walled ureter ("rim sign") around the stone.

Ultrasound of the Kidneys

Ultrasound of the kidneys is performed by scanning the kidney in the longitudinal and transverse planes. The longest axis of the kidney is obtained and measured (Fig. 1–7*A*). Three to six longitudinal images and three transverse images of each kidney are obtained. A normal right kidney should be less echogenic than the adjacent liver at the same depth. A kidney that is more echogenic than the liver is abnormal, but this is a nonspecific finding that may imply many types of renal disease (Fig. 1–7*B*). At ultrasound, the normal kidneys should be between 9 and 13 cm, although allowances are made for body size. Renal sinus fat is hyperechoic and produces a characteristic "central echo complex."

Medullary pyramids in the kidney are usually more hypoechoic than the adjacent renal cortex, especially in newborns (Fig. 1–7). This finding may be confused with hydronephrosis in newborn kidneys. Sinus fat is echogenic in the central portion of the kidney. Mild separation of the walls of the renal pelvis is a normal finding. Emptying of the bladder may sometimes cause this finding to disappear. A separation of the walls of the renal pelvis of greater than 0.5 cm is considered abnormal and implies hydronephrosis.

Doppler ultrasound of an interlobar renal artery to evaluate blood flow allows calculation of a resistive index. The resistive index (RI) is the peak systolic velocity minus the end diastolic velocity divided by the peak systolic velocity. An RI value greater than 0.70 is abnormal and implies low diastolic flow. This may be referred to as a high-resistance pattern. It has been reported that an RI value greater than 0.70 implies abnormality and is useful in separating an obstructed system from a system that is dilated but not obstructed. In our experience, this parameter has not been particularly useful. An elevated RI value will occur anytime something is wrong with the kidney.

Magnetic Resonance Imaging

Magnetic resonance imaging (MRI) of the kidneys is most useful for the evaluation of renal masses. A T1-weighted image usually has a TR (Time of Repetition) of 400 to 800 ms and a TE (Time of Echo) of 5 to 30 ms. These parameters are noted on each image.

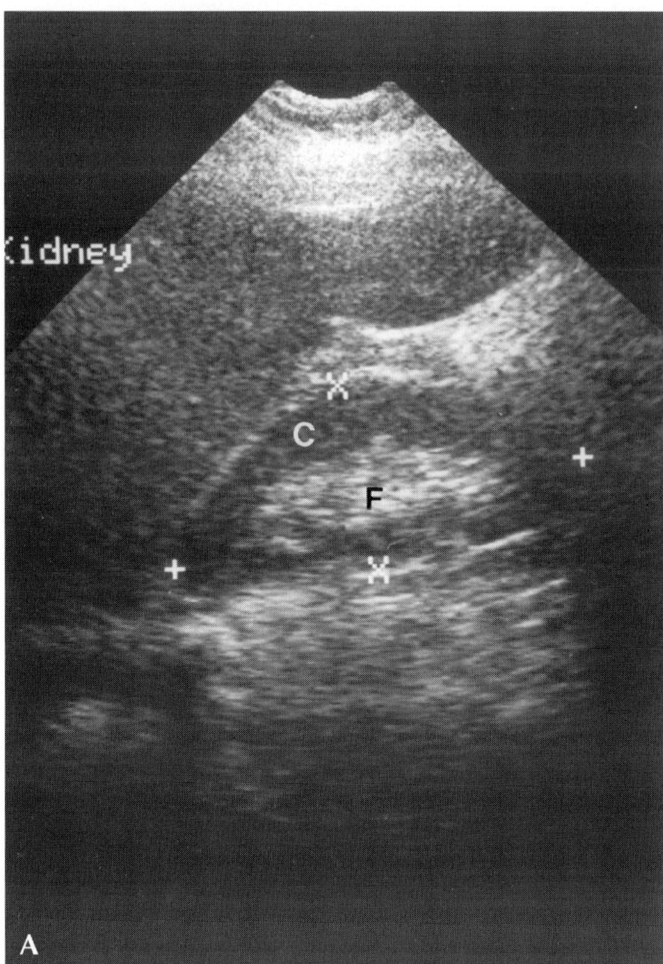

Figure 1–7. A. An ultrasound image of a normal kidney. The kidney is demarcated by + and x. The cortex (C) is less echogenic than the adjacent liver. Renal sinus fat (F) is echogenic. The medullary pyramids are not well seen. **B.** A sagittal ultrasound image of the right kidney showing increased echogenicity in comparison to the adjacent liver (L).

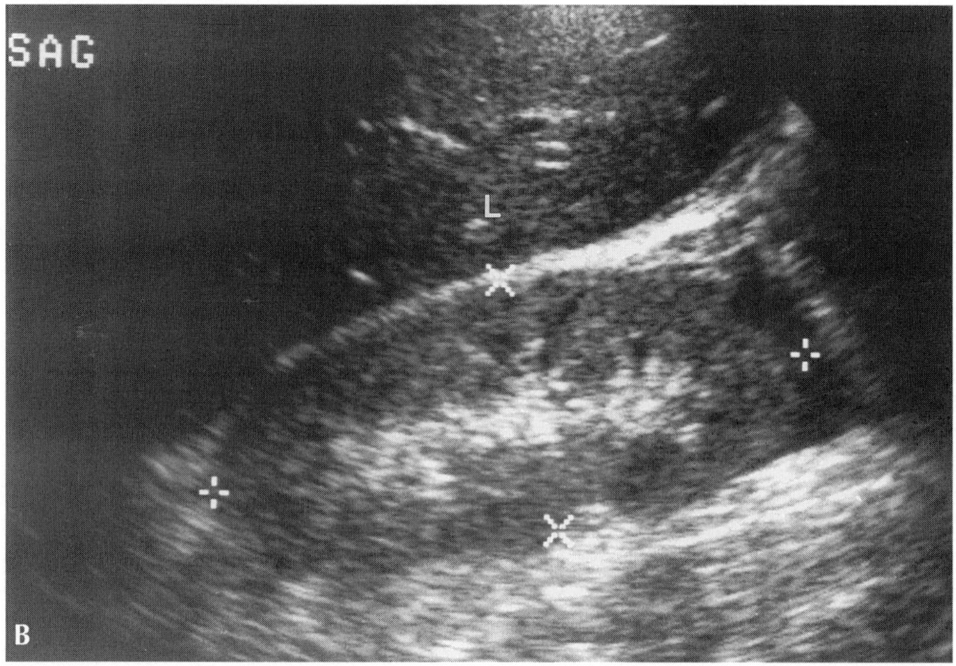

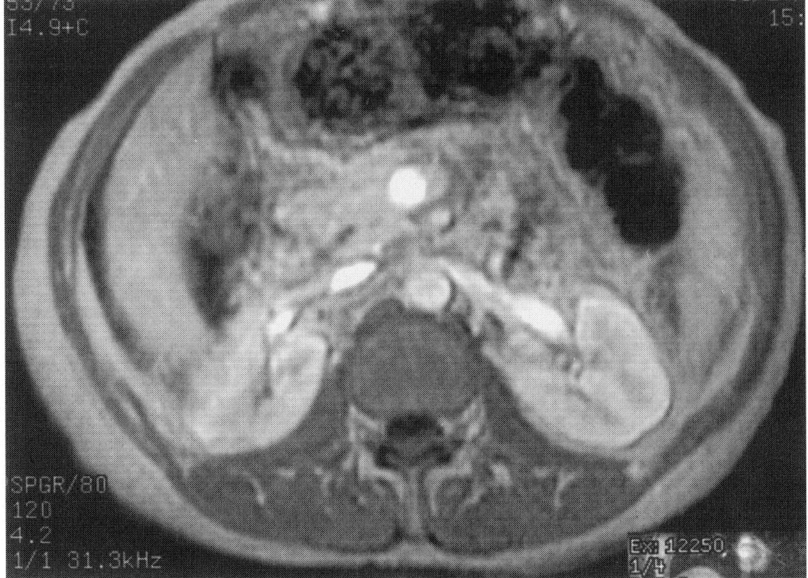

Figure 1–8. An MRI of the kidneys. (A T1-weighted gradient echo breath-hold image.) The cortex is intermediate in signal intensity; the medullary pyramids are dark.

In particular, MRI can be used to identify intracaval extension of renal cell carcinoma. It is also helpful to evaluate renal vein thrombosis. To rule out extension of renal cell carcinoma into the inferior vena cava, sagittal and axial images of the inferior vena cava are obtained. We often use cardiac gating in an effort to create a flow void in the normal inferior vena cava. On an MRI scan, T1-weighted images and T2-weighted images are usually obtained. On a T1-weighted image, water and fluid will usually be of a low signal (dark) and fat will have a high signal (bright). On a T2-weighted image, water will have a higher signal. The normal kidney usually shows low-signal medullary pyramids on T1 images but high-signal ones on T2 images. Magnetic resonance imaging is also used to create angiograms of the aorta and renal arteries. It is valuable in evaluating renal artery stenosis and in evaluating renal transplant donors. Some radiologists prefer gradient echo images (Fig. 1–8). These may be either T1 or T2 weighted. With this type of imaging flowing blood will be bright white.

Retrograde Pyelogram

Retrograde pyelography is performed by the retrograde injection of contrast material through a catheter inserted into the ureteric orifice during cystoscopy of the bladder (Fig. 1–9). The catheter may be advanced to the distal ureter or renal pelvis for injection. The technique is used to determine a cause for hydronephrosis due to ureteric obstruction, especially in patients with impaired ability to excrete contrast material. It is also used to evaluate filling defects in the collecting system when antegrade urography has not sufficiently visualized such defects. If the pelvis and calyces are overdistended by the injection of contrast material, extravasation of contrast material may occur into the veins, lymphatics, or renal sinus (Fig. 1–10). This is referred to as pyelovenous, pyelolymphatic, or pyelosinus backflow, respectively. Calyces will appear more blunted on a retrograde study because of the higher pressures used to distend the pelvis compared to an intravenous pyelogram (IVP). For this reason, the retrograde pyelogram is not a good study for diagnosing hydronephrosis. A drainage film may help to discern the level of obstruction and hydronephrosis. In this situation the collecting system fails to empty.

Nuclear Medicine Renography

Nuclear medicine techniques are used to evaluate the physiology of the kidneys.

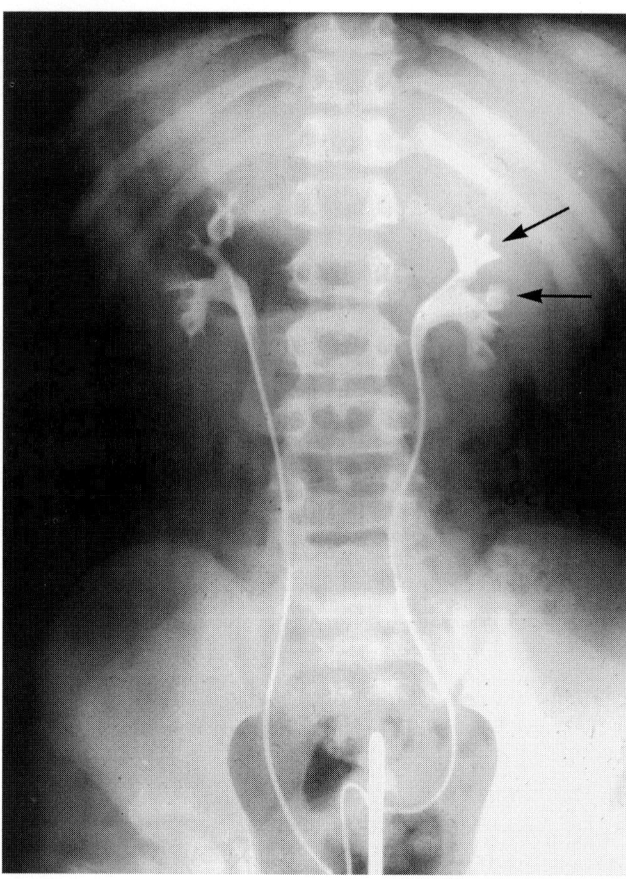

Figure 1–9. This retrograde pyelogram shows injection of both collecting systems. There is a slight blunting of the left calyces (arrows). This is common on retrograde studies because the pressure of injection deforms the collecting system.

They are much less useful for anatomic evaluation. For nuclear renal scanning, a radioactive isotope is attached to a molecule, which is excreted in the urine. These isotopes are usually iodine-123, iodine-131, or preferably technetium-99m. Technetium-99m is preferred because it has superior imaging characteristics and results in less radiation exposure to the patient. Technetium-99m may be attached to diethylenetriamine pentaacetic acid (DTPA). Technetium-99m DTPA is excreted almost completely by glomerular filtration and works quite well in a patient with normal renal function. If the patient has renal impairment, then technetium-99m mercaptoacetyltriglycine (technetium-99m MAG 3) is a better imaging agent. This more expensive radioisotope has a higher rate of clearance from the blood due to a combination of both glomerular filtration and tubular secretion. Technetium-99m glucoheptenate is an older radionuclide that is excreted very slowly by the kidney because it is protein bound. It, and a second radioisotope, technetium-99m dimercaptosuccinic acid (DMSA) are used for anatomic imaging to determine whether a lesion in the kidney is a functioning or nonfunctioning tissue (implying that it is a renal cell carcinoma). This test has fallen from favor and has largely been replaced by CT scanning, but it may be useful to exclude a column of Bertin.

Both technetium-99m DTPA and MAG 3 are administered as a bolus. Images of the kidneys are obtained every 1 to 3 seconds for about 1 minute to allow evaluation of renal perfusion. Images are then obtained every 2 to 5 minutes for approximately 30 minutes. A normal perfusion study will show peak activity in the kidneys within 6 seconds of the aortic peak. Delay of the peak implies impaired perfusion. Following the peak, a washout of the radionuclide from the kidneys should occur. Progressive accumulation of the radionuclide is abnormal. Delayed images (Fig. 1–11) should also show a peak in cortical activity by 5 min-

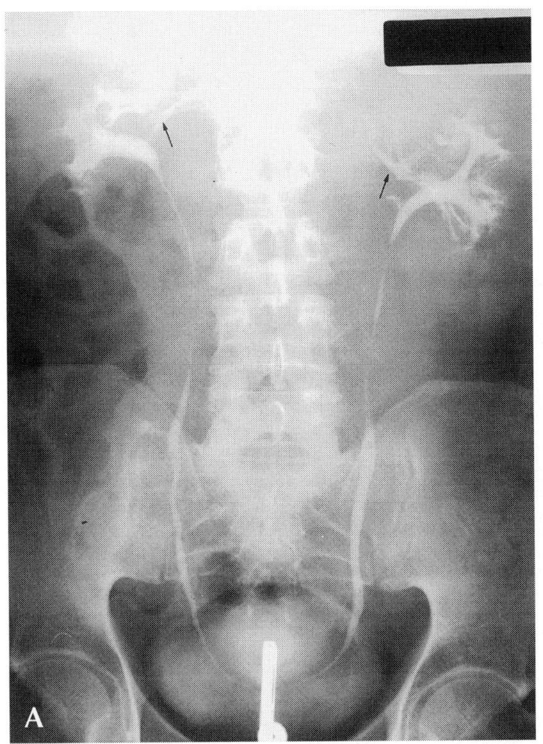

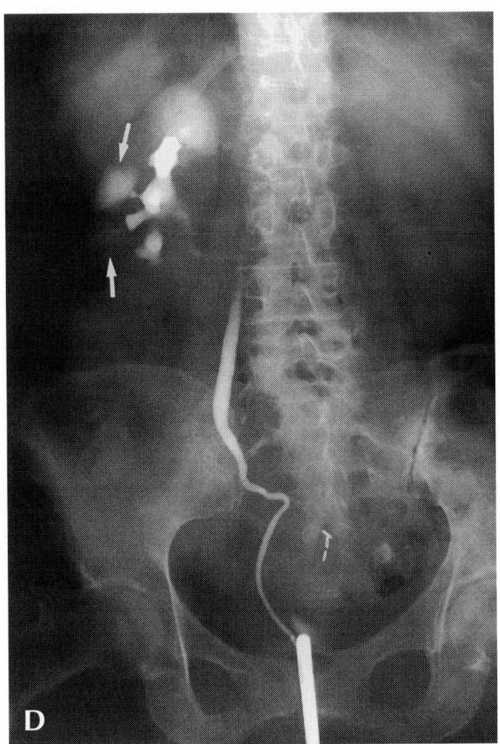

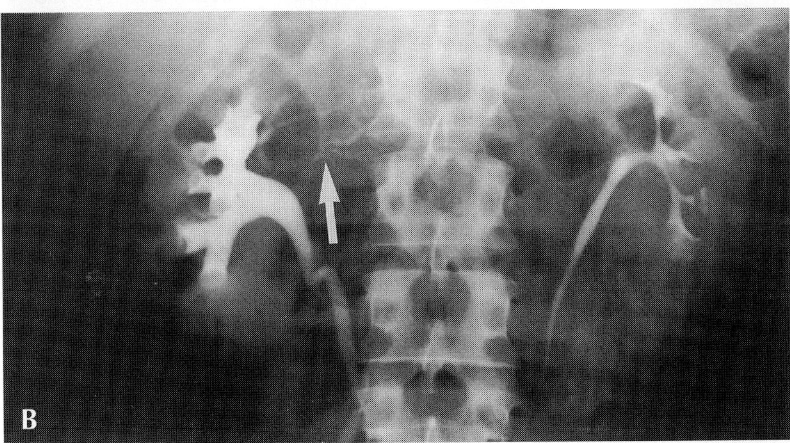

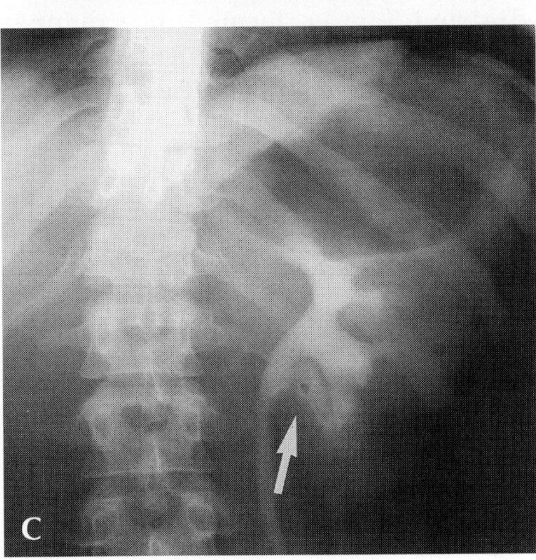

Figure 1–10. A. Pyelovenous backflow. Forceful injection of contrast material leads to contrast material in veins (arrows). **B.** Pyelolymphotic backflow. Sometimes the high-pressure injection results in contrast material being carried away by lymphatics (arrows). These are more squiggly than veins. **C.** Pyelosinus backflow. Contrast material has entered the area of the renal sinus (arrow). **D.** Pyelotubular backflow. There is reflux into the distal collecting tubules (arrow).

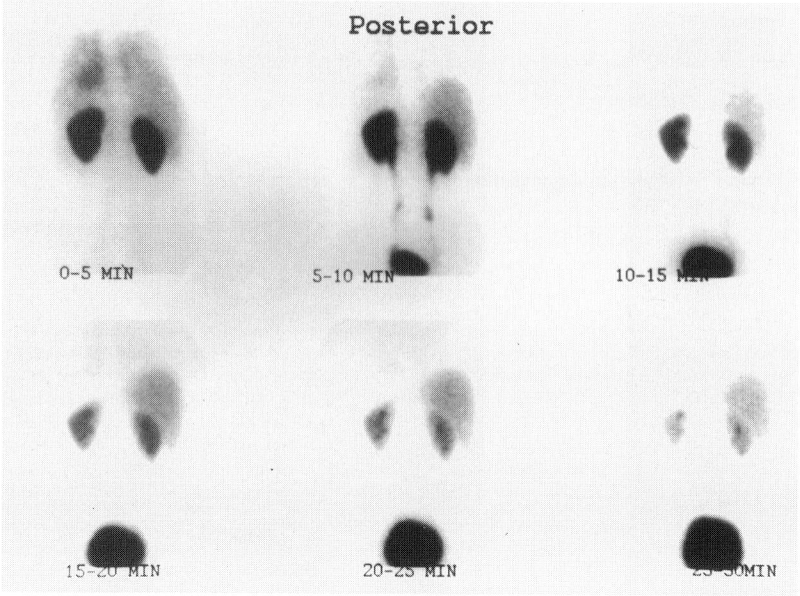

Figure 1–11. Posterior images of a normal technetium-99m MAG 3 renogram. There is a peak in renal activity by 5 minutes and rapid washout.

utes, implying that the kidney can promptly extract the radionuclide from the blood. Impairment in the function of the kidney may be inferred if the peak occurs later than 5 minutes. A visual washout of activity should occur within 10 minutes to a value equal to half the peak level. In normal subjects, activity should be identifiable within the collecting system by that time as well.

To evaluate hydronephrosis, lasix may be administered approximately 15 or 20 minutes into this exam at the time of peak cortical activity. A region of interest is placed around the kidney by computer, and the counts of radioactivity are measured in the kidney as a function of time. An obstructed kidney will show progressive accumulation of the radioactivity, whereas a normal nonobstructed kidney will show prompt elimination of the radionuclide after the lasix, with a 50 percent decrease in radioactivity over the first 10 minutes.

Pediatrics

Because the pediatric patient has a reduced glomerular filtration rate up to age 2, higher doses of contrast material must be administered (Table 1–2). In the pediatric patient, the intravenous urogram may be performed in a more abbreviated fashion than in an adult. Usually the kidneys, ureters, and bladder are more easily visualized due to reduced body mass. We obtain an immediate film after the injection of contrast and a 10-minute film. Any other films are tailored to the clinical problem.

Renal ultrasound in the pediatric patient is similar to that in adults. In the neonate, the cortex of the kidney is more echogenic than it is in an adult. The echogenicity of the kidney cortex will often equal that of the liver and may occasionally be greater. In the neonate the medullary pyramids appear more prominent simply because the contrast between the medullary pyramids and the echogenic renal cortex is greater (Fig. 1–12).

Pediatric CT is performed in a manner similar to the scanning of adults. However, the slice thickness may be reduced to 5 mm in smaller patients.

NORMAL VARIANTS

Column of Bertin

A column of Bertin is a normal variant in which renal cortex extends between the medullary pyramids (Fig. 1–13). Columns of Bertin are more common if there is duplica-

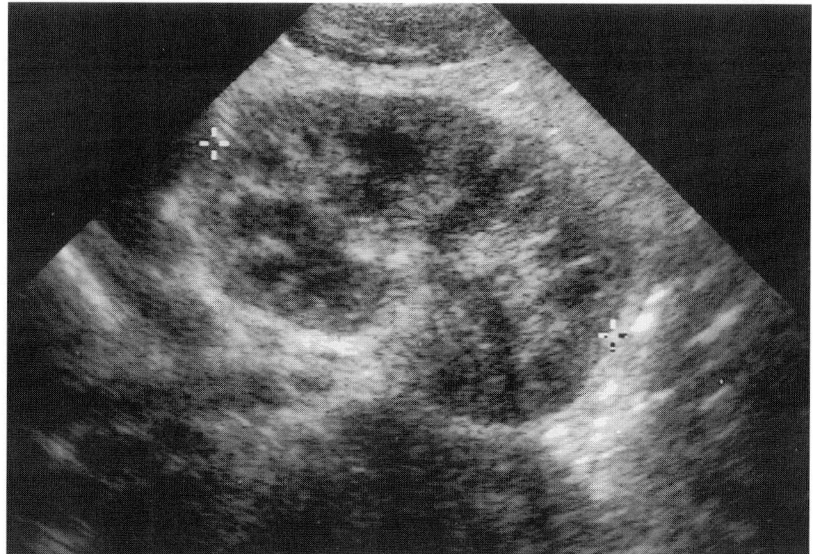

Figure 1–12. A sagittal image of a normal neonatal kidney. The cortex is more echogenic and the medullary pyramids are more echolucent than in an adult.

tion. These columns may be bulbous in appearance, creating a pseudotumor appearance. A column of Bertin may cause displacement of the collecting system on intravenous urography. On ultrasound, the tissue that projects into the medullary portion of the kidney can simulate a mass. This problem can be solved with a contrast-enhanced CT scan or radionuclide imaging. Columns of Bertin enhance on CT imaging in the normal fashion, indicating that functioning nephrons are present. Likewise, there should be normal accumulation of radioisotope on nuclear imaging. The most commonly used radioisotopes for this purpose are technetium-99m glucoheptonate and technetium-99m DMSA.

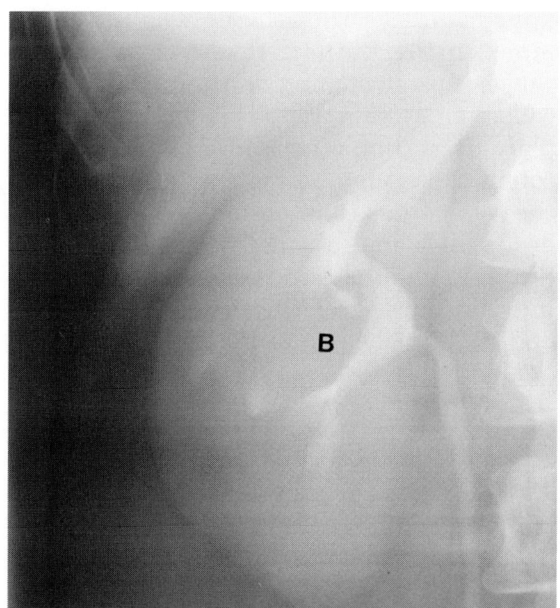

Figure 1–13. An intravenous urogram. The column of Bertin (B) extends into the medullary portion of the kidney and splays the collecting system.

Splenic Compression

The lateral superior margin of the left kidney may be flattened with a bulge at the midportion. This unusual shape is caused by molding of the renal contour by the adjacent spleen. The bulge is often referred to as a "dromedary hump" (Fig. 1–2). The thickness of the cortex should be uniform when measured from each calyx to adjoining cortex. Computed tomography or radionuclide studies can be performed to confirm that the bulge is normally functioning renal tissue and that it is not a tumor.

Vascular Impressions

Vascular impressions occur when arteries or veins compress the pelvocalyceal system or ureter (Fig. 1–14). These may be either nor-

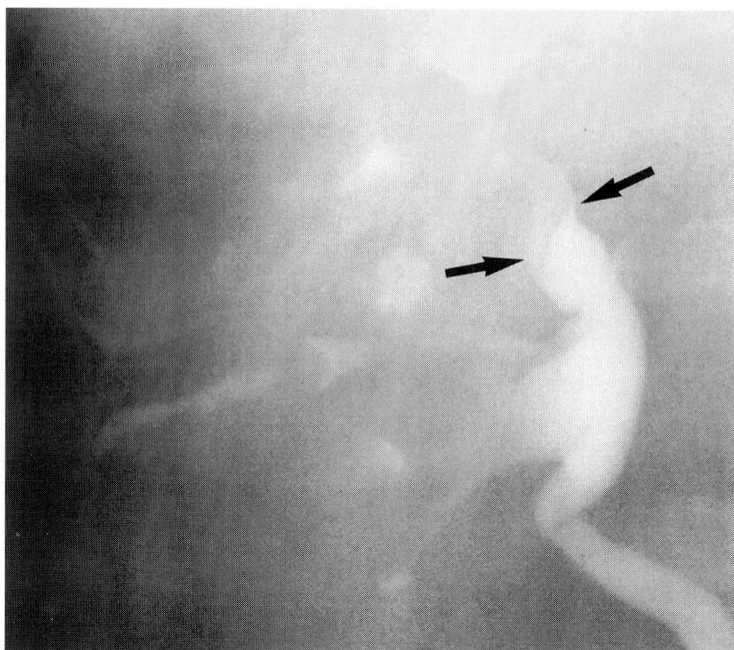

Figure 1–14. An intravenous urogram. The crossing vessel causes an impression (arrows) on the upper-pole infundibulum.

mal or aberrant vessels. Impressions caused by arteries are more common than those caused by veins because of the higher pressures in arteries. Vascular impressions are very common in the infundibulum to the upper-pole calyx and appear as a smooth line that bisects, or partially bisects, the infundibular tissue. If an impression is caused by a vessel, then a change in patient position may cause a change in the size of the impression or its orientation.

Renal Sinus Lipomatosis

Renal sinus lipomatosis is a term used to describe an excess of fat in the renal sinus. Fat is normally found in this location. In obese and older individuals, there is usually an increase in the amount of this fat. Renal sinus fat can be increased further by processes that lead to destruction of the kidney as when fat replaces renal mass that is lost. On urography, the collecting system may be stretched and have an appearance as though there is a central mass in the kidney. However, when fat causes this stretching or attenuation of the collecting system, the fat is more lucent on plain films than other soft tissue. On ultrasound there may be more echogenic fat in the renal sinus than normal. A CT scan can be used to make a definitive diagnosis. Sinus lipomatosis can also cause stretching and bowing of the main renal artery and its branches on either CT scanning or angiography.

Chapter

2

Upper Tract Congenital Anomalies

CALYCEAL DIVERTICULA

Calyceal diverticula (Fig. 2–1) can originate either from the calyx or from the renal pelvis. Because of this, they are more accurately called pyelocalyceal diverticula. They occur in both sexes and are sometimes classified as Type I and Type II diverticula. Type I diverticula usually communicate with the calyx at the fornix. They are spherical in shape, may occur at the lower pole (but more commonly arise from the upper pole), and have a narrow connecting stalk. Type II diverticula are located more centrally, are larger, have a shorter neck, and communicate with the renal pelvis.

Two theories explain the formation of these diverticula. Embryologically, they may represent ureteral bud remnants that have not fully formed into calyces. A second theory holds that calyceal diverticula are acquired due to chronic reflux or infection involving either the calyx itself or an adjacent renal cyst. Ultimately, a communication develops with the calyx. About 50 percent of patients will form stones within the diverticulum. They may also form milk of calcium, which is a supersaturated or colloidal suspension of calcium salts and appears as a radiopaque density on plain films with a fluid calcium level. Symptoms result from infection or stones within the diverticulum. Since diverticula are lined by transitional epithelium, transitional cell carcinoma may develop.

During the intravenous urogram, the diverticulum should opacify, but the opacification may be delayed due to slow exchange of fluid between the calyx and the diverticulum. On ultrasound and CT scan, the diverticula appear as cystic water density lesions unless there are stones or milk of calcium within. A distinction between these lesions and simple cysts may be impossible on ultrasound and CT scan unless the lesion opacifies with the administration of intravenous contrast material or stones move with changes in patient position. A calyceal diverticulum may also be confused with focal caliectasis, especially when the caliectasis is due to infundibular narrowing.

ECTOPIC PELVIC KIDNEY (RENAL ECTOPIA)

Embryologically, the kidneys ascend from the pelvis to the renal fossa. The ureteral bud,

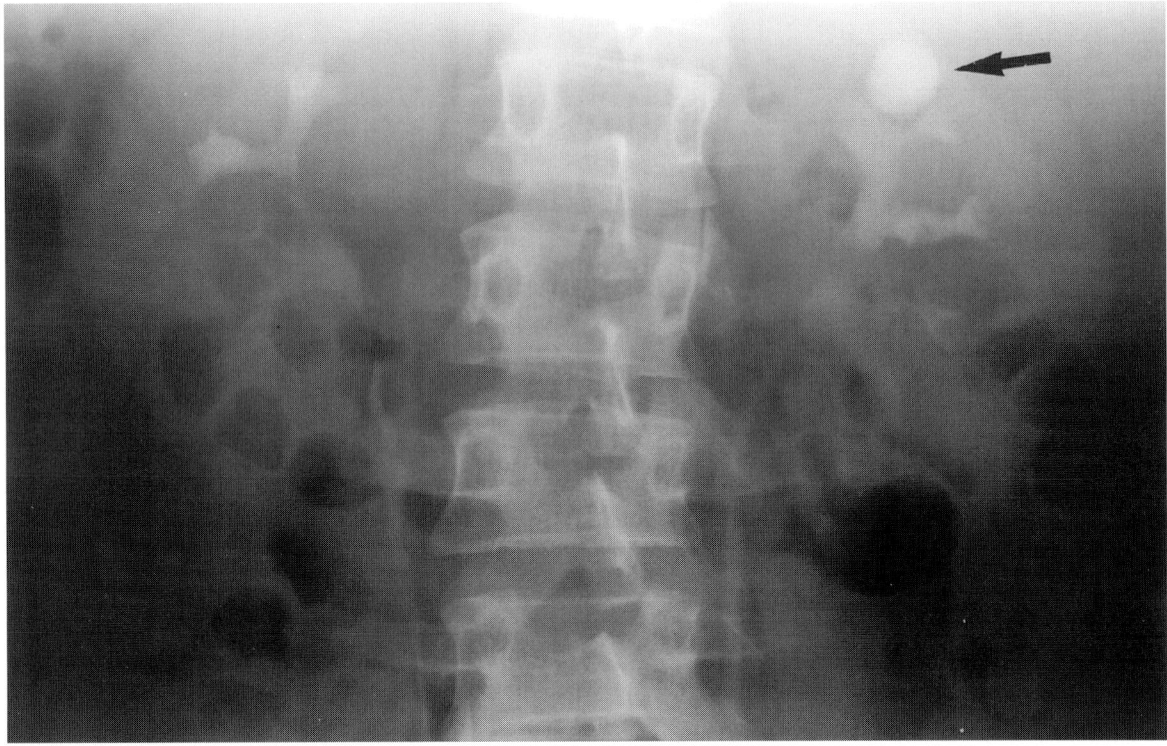

Figure 2–1. A left upper-pole calyceal diverticulum (arrow). This is a type I diverticulum.

arising from the mesonephric duct, elongates during this process. As the kidney ascends it obtains a blood supply from more cephalad portions of the aorta. If ureteral bud elongation or acquisition of new blood supply is abnormal or there is a physical barrier to cephalad migration, the kidney may come to occupy an abnormal position. Ectopic kidneys are frequently located in the pelvis (Fig. 2–2*A–D*). Fifty percent of these pelvic kidneys have associated hydronephrosis or vesicoureteral reflux. Occasionally, the kidney may migrate into the thorax to become an intrathoracic kidney. This occurs more commonly on the left than on the right.

On urography, identification of a pelvic kidney depends on how well the kidney is functioning. A pelvic kidney may also be obscured by a large bladder or the bony pelvis. Ultrasound may not be helpful in identifing a pelvic or ectopic kidney when confusion is created by adjacent loops of bowel. An ectopic kidney can almost always be identified by CT scan (Fig. 2–2*C*). Technetium-99m DPTA nuclear medicine scans are also very helpful in locating the kidney. These will often have identifiable activity, even when there is poor renal function (Fig. 2–2*D*).

Occasionally, a ureteral bud may come in contact with the contralateral metanephric ridge. This leads to a condition known as cross-fused ectopia. All of the renal mass is located on one side of the abdomen, but the distal ureter crosses the midline to insert in the bladder at the appropriate location. This condition is more common in children with myelodysplasia.

PERSISTENT FETAL URETER

Ureteral valves or persistent fetal ureter occurs due to persistence of the physiologic folds seen in ureters of fetuses and neonates. Clinically, the presentation is usually incidental. Radiographically, on either antegrade or retrograde pyelography the ureter shows a beaded or corkscrew appearance without hydronephrosis.

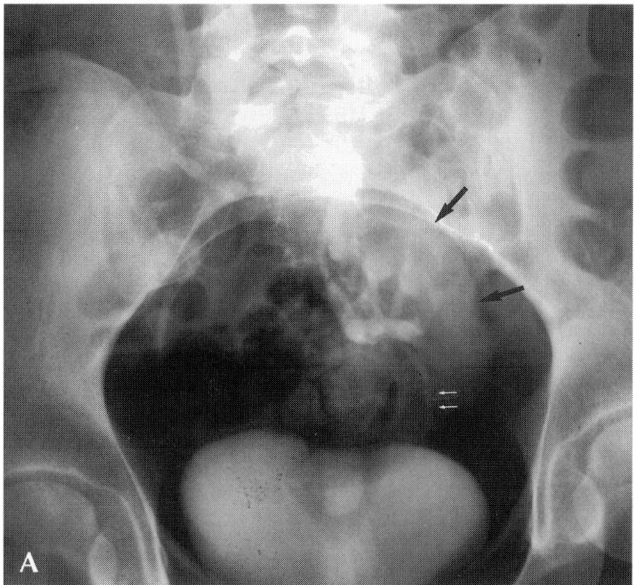

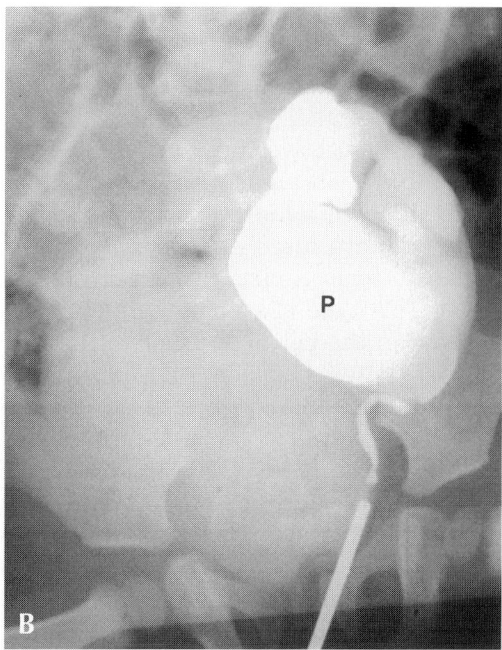

Figure 2–2. A. A pelvic kidney. The kidney is outlined by arrows. The small arrows point to the ureter. **B.** Retrograde pyelography in a different patient shows filling of the dilated renal pelvis (P) of a pelvic kidney. **C.** CT scan of a patient with pelvic kidney (K). **D.** This posterior image from a nuclear medicine study shows activity in the right kidney (R) and in the pelvic left kidney (arrow).

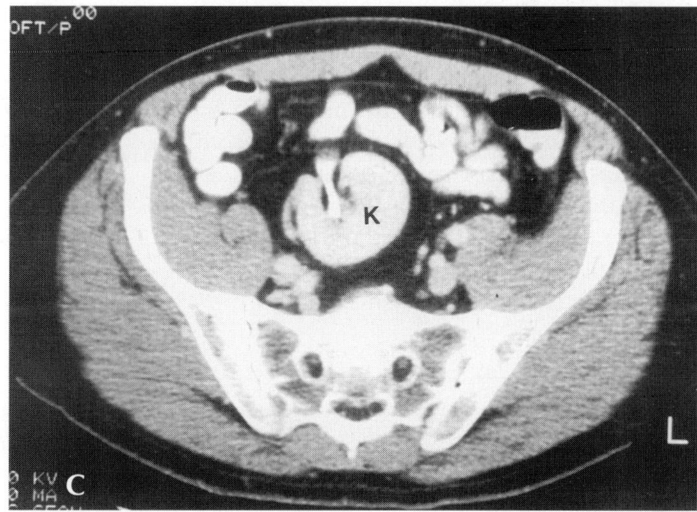

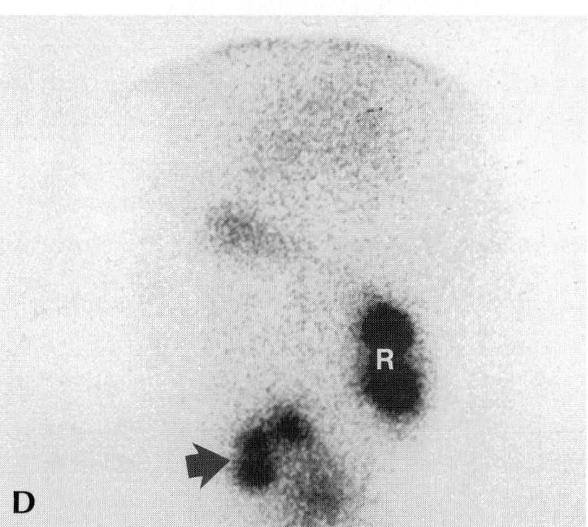

FUSION ANOMALIES

"Disk," "pancake," "lump," "cake," and "horseshoe" are adjectives used to describe various forms of fusion anomalies. The disk or pancake kidney is a kidney that has the left and right kidneys fused at the upper and lower poles to form a circular renal mass (Fig. 2–3). This type of ectopic kidney is usually located in the pelvis anterior to the sacrum. Ureters enter the bladder normally.

Horseshoe kidneys are fused in the midline at the lower poles of the right and left kidneys (Fig. 2–4). The attachment may simply be a band of fibrous tissue or functional renal tissue. Horseshoe kidneys usually lie in a more caudal location than normal. The renal pelves and collecting systems are malrotated anteriorly. They frequently have multiple aberrant renal arteries. The lower poles are often fused at a level caudal to the inferior mesenteric artery. The perirenal space of each kidney communicates across the midline. About one-third of horseshoe kidneys have an associated ureteropelvic junction (UPJ) obstruction. One-third of these patients also have other congenital anomalies, including gastrointestinal, cardiovascular, and skeletal malformations. These kidneys may be more prone to damage at the time of abdominal trauma, and there may be an increased incidence of malignancy.

Because of the lower-pole fusion, horseshoe kidneys have an abnormal axis and the lower poles are deviated medially. A key identifying feature on urography is a medially directed calyx (Fig. 2–4*A*). On ultrasound examination it may be difficult to appreciate that a horseshoe kidney is present because the connecting isthmus may not be identifiable. On CT scan, this isthmus can often be seen and anterior orientation of the renal hilum is more obvious (Fig. 2–4*B*).

URETERAL DUPLICATION

With ureteral duplication, two ureteral buds branch independently from the mesonephric duct and fuse with metanephric blastema. This produces two complete collecting systems, and two ureters drain the ipsilateral renal unit (Fig. 2–5*A*). The lower-pole ureter usually drains the lower two-thirds of the kidney, and the orifice is located superiolaterally to the upper-pole orifice in the bladder. The ureter that drains the upper-pole

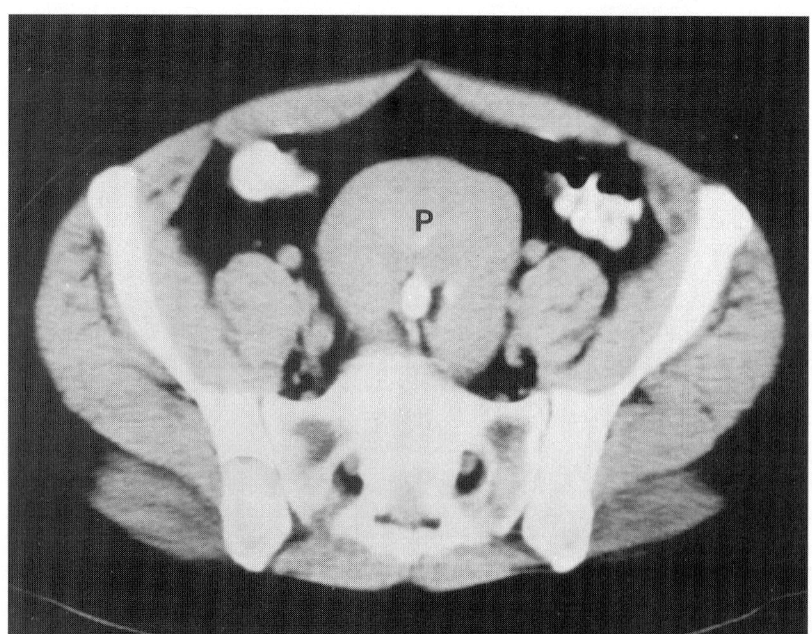

Figure 2–3. Pancake kidney (P).

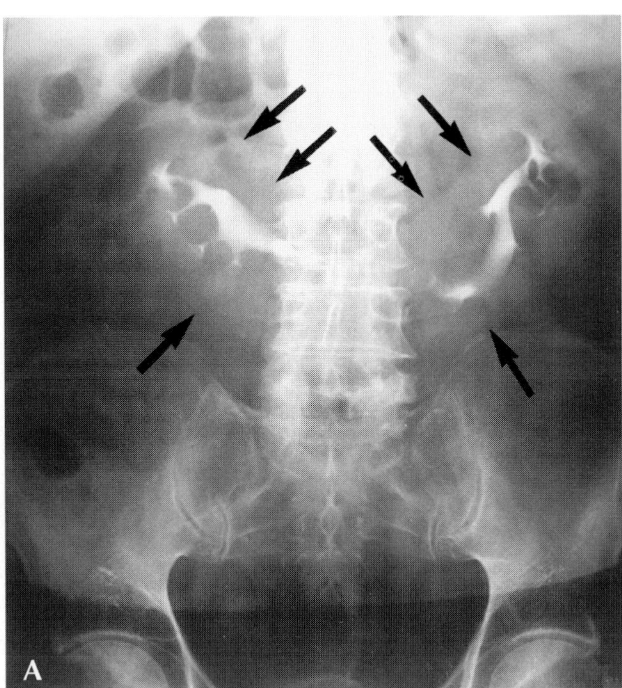

Figure 2–4. A. Intravenous urography (IVU). The kidneys are outlined by arrows. The lower poles are fused and deviate medially. **B.** A CT scan in a different patient shows fused lower poles (F).

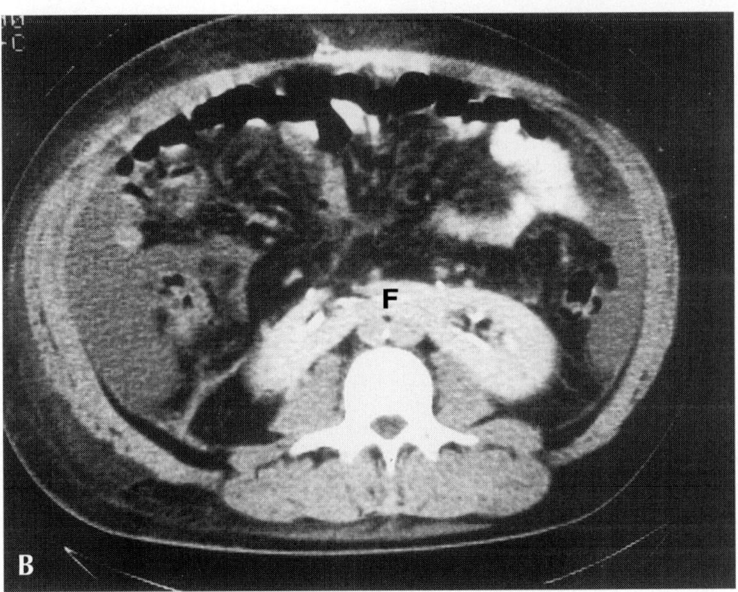

segment usually drains a smaller renal mass and enters the bladder medially and inferior to the lower-pole orifice. The upper-pole orifice may enter the urinary tract ectopically and is more commonly obstructed. Ectopic insertion may be associated with a ureterocele. The lower-pole ureter is subject to reflux because of a lateral location on the trigone and a short intramural segment. Duplicated kidneys are larger than nonduplicated kidneys.

Partial duplications are much more common (Fig. 2–5*B*). For partial duplications two ureters merge and there is only one urinary insertion site into the bladder. Partial duplications are less likely to have clinical symptoms. A phenomenon known as "yo-yo" peristalsis has been described in which the peristaltic wave from one ureter travels up the other, leading to renorenal reflux. The clinical significance of this phenomenon is unclear.

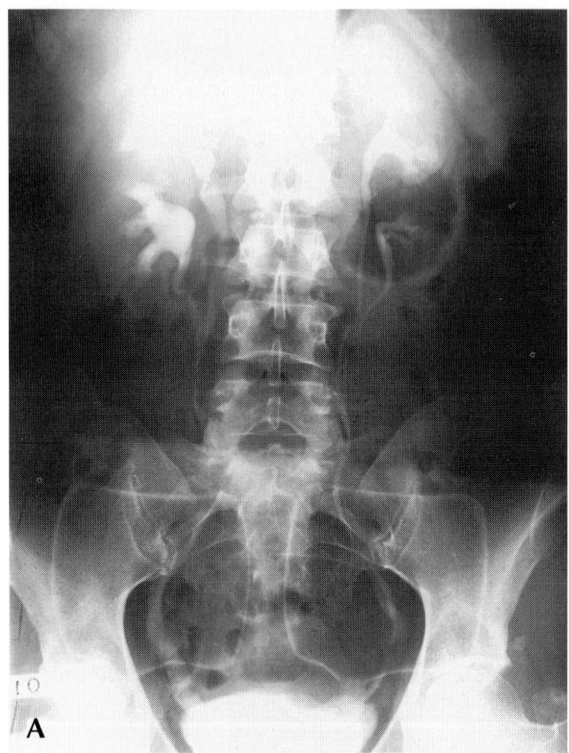

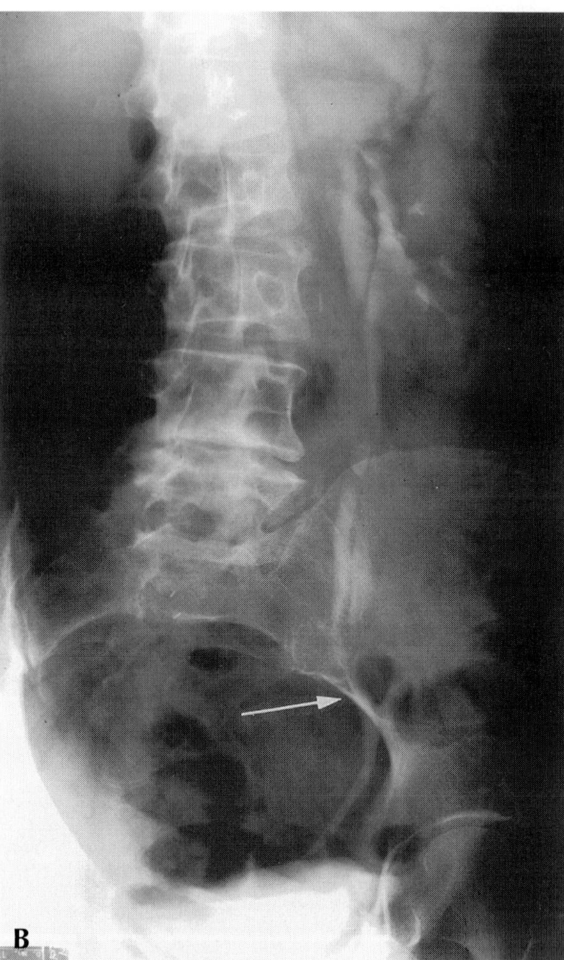

Figure 2–5. A. Bilateral duplicated collecting systems. There are two pelves and two ureters draining each kidney. **B.** Partial duplication of the left kidney. There are two pelves and two ureters, but the ureters merge into one at the lower end of the SI joint (arrow).

At intravenous pyelography, two ureters and two renal pelves may be identified. Dilatation of either ureter may be present, although the upper-pole ureter will more likely be dilated. Severe obstruction may obviate visualization of the upper-pole moiety. The term *drooping lily* has been used at urography to denote hydronephrosis of the upper pole that is pushing the lower pole calyces in a downward direction, leading to the appearance of a drooping flower (Fig. 2–6*A*). Delayed films may allow opacification of the upper-pole portion so that the diagnosis can be made.

An ectopic ureter is a ureter that does not terminate in the trigone of the bladder in the usual location. However, the term is usually used to denote a ureter that empties outside of the bladder. Ectopic ureters are most commonly associated with the upper-pole segment of a complete duplication of the collecting system in females. In males, it is more common for the ectopic ureter to drain a nonduplicated system. Development of the trigone of the bladder reflects whether or not a ureter inserts in the appropriate location. If no ureter inserts into the bladder, there will also be inadequate development of the ipsilateral trigone in the bladder. In females, the ureteral orifice insertion may open into the uterus, vagina, cervix, bladder neck, vestibule, or urethra. In males, insertion may occur into the bladder neck, prostatic urethra, seminal vesicles, vas

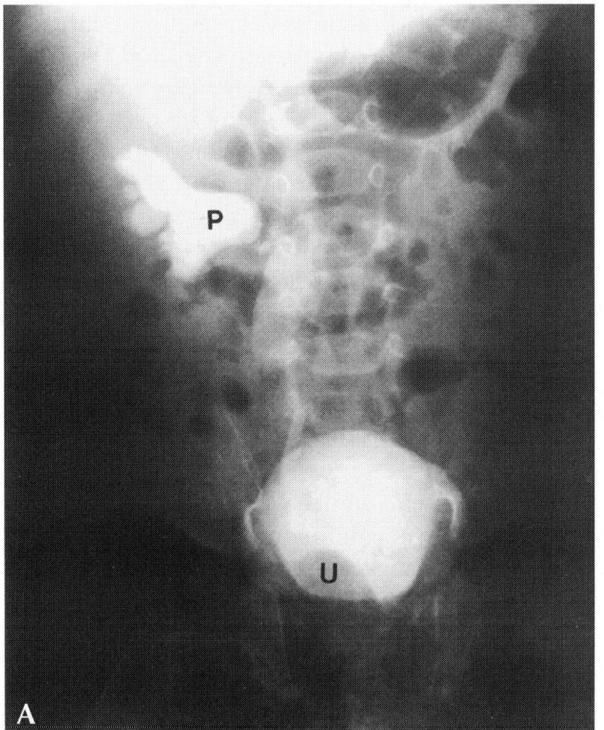

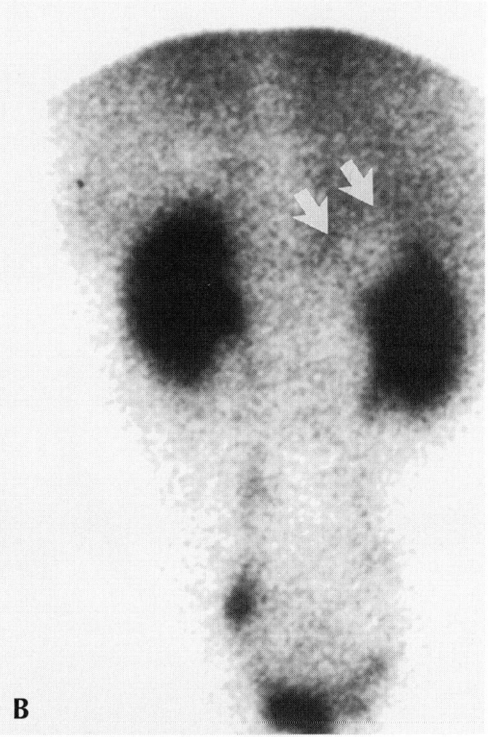

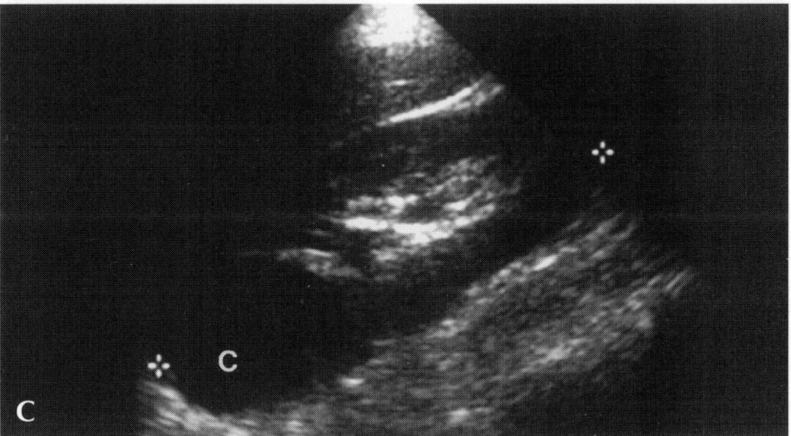

Figure 2–6. A. Here the lower-pole collecting system (P) is pushed inferiorly by the nonopacified hydronephrotic upper-pole collecting system. A large ureterocele (U) causes a filling defect in the bladder. **B.** A posterior image from a nuclear medicine study showing a void (arrows) where the nonfunctioning hydronephrotic right upper-pole duplication is located. **C.** A coronal ultrasound image of the right kidney showing a dilated upper-pole collecting system (C).

deferens, or ejaculatory duct. Ectopic ureters present clinically with infection and obstruction with stone formation (Fig. 2–7). In females, continuous incontinence with an otherwise normal voiding pattern may result if the ectopic ureter inserts distal to the sphincter. When associated with a duplicated collecting system, the orifice of the ectopic ureter is often stenotic, leading to obstruction of the upper-pole segment.

Vesicoureteral reflux into an ectopic upper-pole segment and a laterally placed

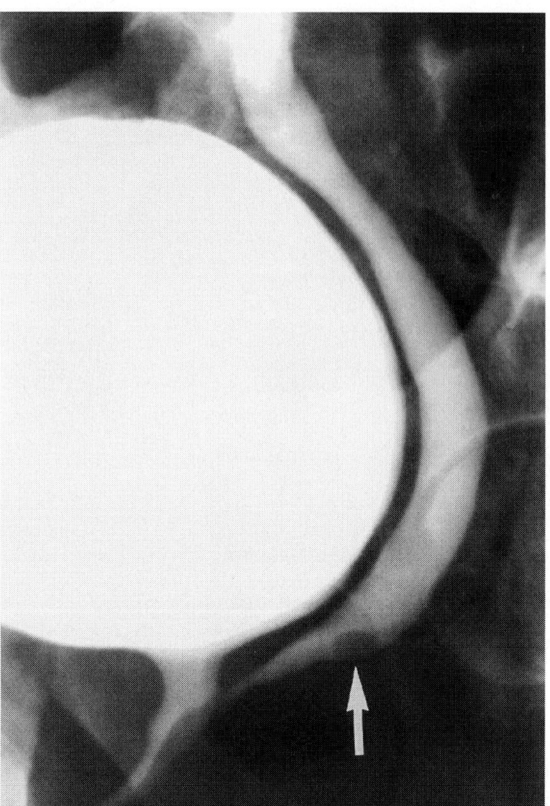

Figure 2–7. An ectopic ureter inserts into this urethra with a distal uric acid stone (arrow).

lower-pole segment may be demonstrated at the time of voiding cystourethrography. Reflux into an associated ureterocele is uncommon but may be seen with large cecoureteroceles. A cecoureterocele has a long tongue of ureterocele extending distal to the bladder neck. The orifice is in the bladder and is patulous. Long-standing vesicoureteral reflux may result in marked scarring and deformity of the lower pole of the kidney. On renal ultrasound, there may be two distinct clumps of echogenic fat in the renal sinuses. It may not be possible to distinguish a partial or complete duplication with this ultrasound unless there is evidence of dilatation of the renal pelvis, calyces, or upper ureter for the upper- or lower-pole moieties. It may be more difficult to appreciate duplication on CT scan unless two ureters can be clearly identified. A cut through the midportion of the kidney that does not show any renal sinus fat can be suggestive of duplication. Ureteroceles are congenital or acquired cystic dilatations of the ureter, most often associated with the upper-pole ureter of duplication. The orifice draining a ureterocele may be orthotopic or ectopic. Orthotopic or "simple" ureteroceles are ureteroceles appearing in the ureter in the normal location. These are usually incidental findings in adults. A stone may form in the lumen of a ureterocele (Fig. 2–8*A*).

Ectopic ureteroceles are more common in females and duplicated systems. They may present with urinary tract infection or obstructed bladder outlet due to prolapse of the ureterocele through the urethra. Occasionally, a ureterocele may be so large as to obstruct the orifice of the contralateral ureter, or, by deforming the contralateral trigone of a normally inserted ureter, may cause reflux.

At urography, a simple ureterocele may appear as a filling defect in the opacified bladder (Fig. 2–8B). The distal ureter will be slightly dilated. A thin line of lucency, caused by the wall of the distal ureter, separates the dilated ureter from the contrast in the bladder. This is sometimes called a "cobra head" deformity (Fig. 2–8*B*). Ectopic ureteroceles, on the other hand, may produce a large filling defect on an IVP.

URETEROPELVIC JUNCTION OBSTRUCTION

Congenital ureteropelvic junction (UPJ) obstruction is a disorder that is most often detected in infancy or childhood. Diagnosis in the neonate is currently quite common because of the widespread use of obstetric ultrasound in the identification of a dilated renal pelvis in utero. This is not a mechanical obstruction but instead is a functional obstruction. The most common theory postulates a disorder of smooth muscle at the level of the UPJ, leading to interruption of the peristaltic wave as it travels down the renal pelvis into the ureter. An alternate theory states that this portion of the ureter is not distensible due to a disorder of collagen. Rare causes include crossing blood vessels and fibrous bands, which may kink the

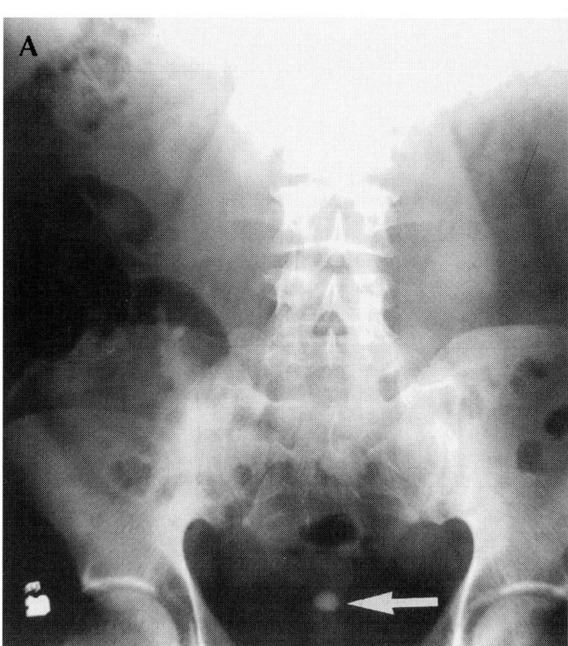

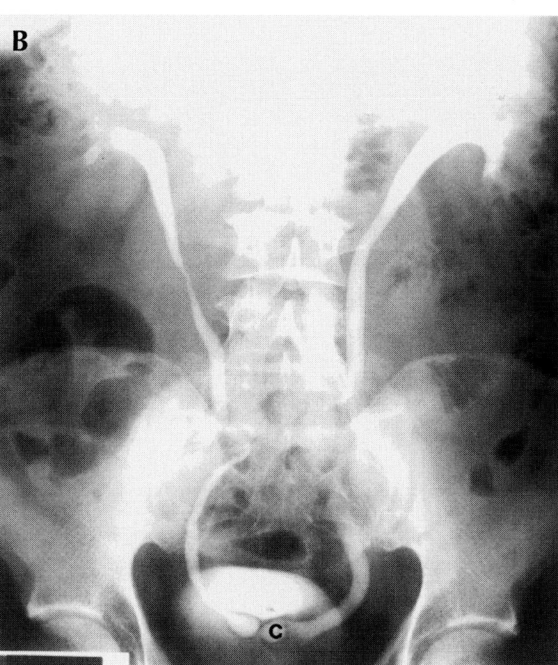

Figure 2–8. A ureterocele. **A.** Plain film shows a calcific density projecting over the sacrum (arrow). **B.** An IVU in the same patient shows that a calcific density projects over the left "cobra head" and represents a stone in the ureterocele.

ureter. Usually the blood vessels in this area are incidental to this diagnosis. UPJ obstruction most often presents as an abdominal mass in neonates, but more commonly presents with urinary tract infection or pain in older children. The left kidney is more often involved. There is a 2:1 ratio between males and females.

On antegrade or retrograde urography, hydronephrosis of the renal pelvis and calyces is seen (Fig. 2–9). There may be slow opacification of the affected side, and it may be necessary to obtain delayed films to be certain that the level of obstruction is truly at the ureteropelvic junction rather than ureterovesical obstruction. In severe cases, there will be cortical thinning with only a rim of functioning cortical parenchyma surrounding a dilated collecting system. The "crescent" sign is seen on IVP or CT scan as a thin rim of contrast pooling in the collecting duct and suggests salvageable function. Hydronephrosis secondary to UPJ obstruction may be massive and may cross the abdominal midline. On ultrasound or CT, findings are simply those of a dilated pelvis and calyces. This dilatation may not be present if the patient is studied while dehydrated. A nuclear medicine study utilizing technetium-99m DPTA with the administration of lasix may be useful to demonstrate that a true obstruction is present. In the newborn, the major differential is between multicystic dysplastic kidney and UPJ obstruction. This distinction can be made with a lasix renogram, which will show absence of blood flow in the event of multicystic dysplastic kidney.

RETROCAVAL URETER

Retrocaval ureter embryologically occurs due to persistence of the subcardinal vein. The right ureter courses posterior to the inferior vena cava at approximately L3 or L4 (Fig. 2–10). Distal to this point, the ureter then begins moving lateral to its normal position. On intravenous urography, retrocaval ureter is in the differential diag-

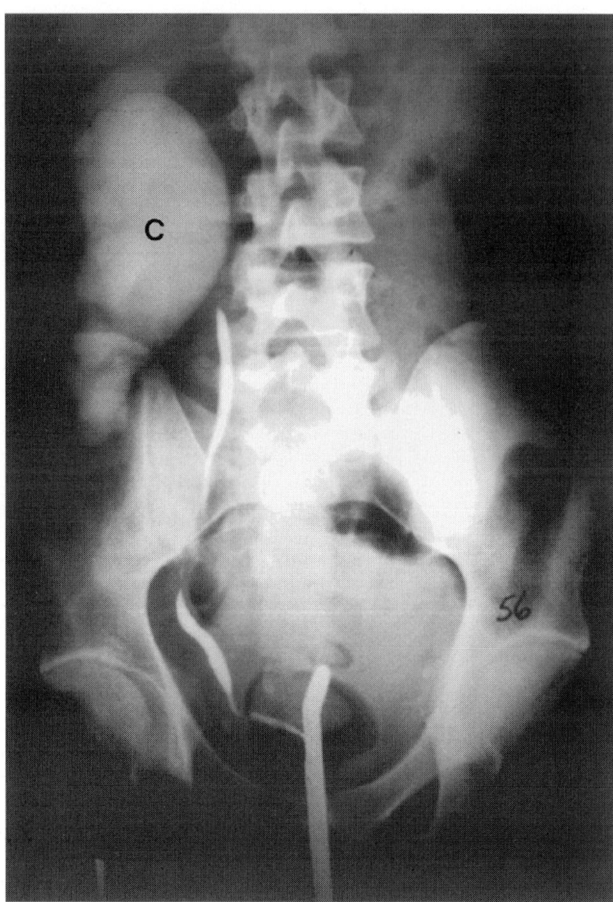

Figure 2–9. This retrograde study shows massive dilatation of the right collecting system (C) in this patient with a UPJ obstruction.

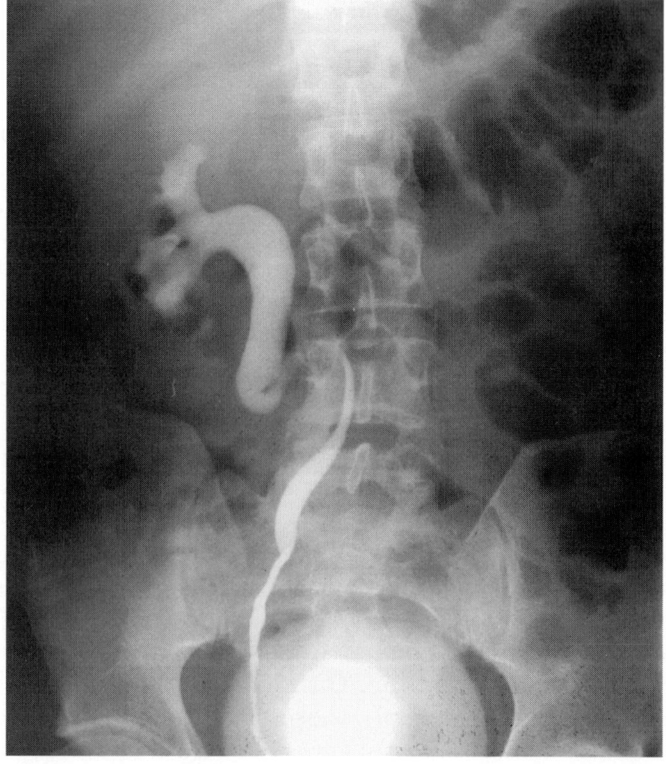

Figure 2–10. Retrocaval ureter. The upper third of the ureter deviates behind the vena cava, where it is partially obstructed.

nosis for obstruction of the right kidney involving the upper third of the ureter. The ureter distal to the obstruction, if seen, is medially deviated. This is frequently an incidental finding at CT. Most often the patients are asymptomatic but may present with flank pain or urinary tract infection.

URETERAL DIVERTICULUM

At approximately 5 weeks' gestational age, a ureteral bud can be identified. This ureteral bud elongates and contacts the metanephric blastema. When this fails to occur there will be a blind-ending ureter without any attachment to the superior pole of the kidney. This is also known as a ureteral diverticulum (Fig. 2–11*A* and *B*).

PRIMARY MEGAURETER

Primary megaureter describes dilatation of the ureter due to causes other than reflux or mechanical obstruction. The anatomical

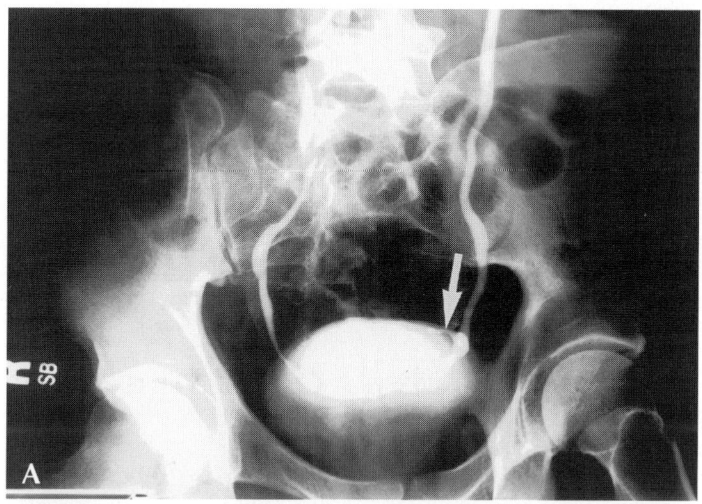

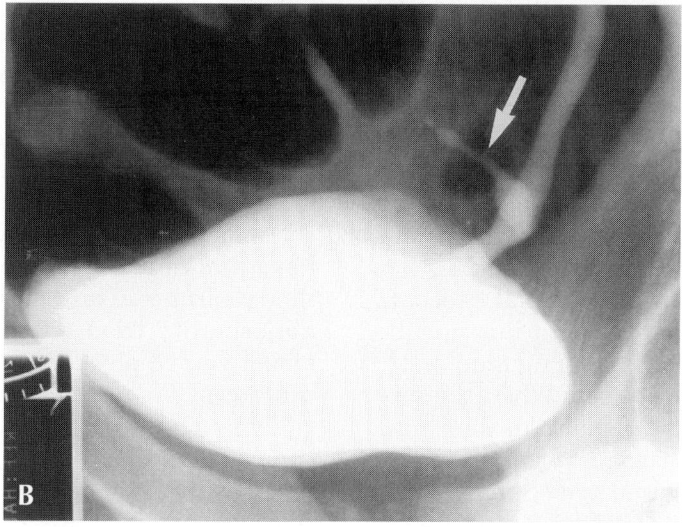

Figure 2–11. A. This film of the pelvis shows a ureteral diverticulum (arrow). Usually these diverticula are found in the proximal ureter. **B.** The coned-down film shows the diverticulum (arrow) in greater detail.

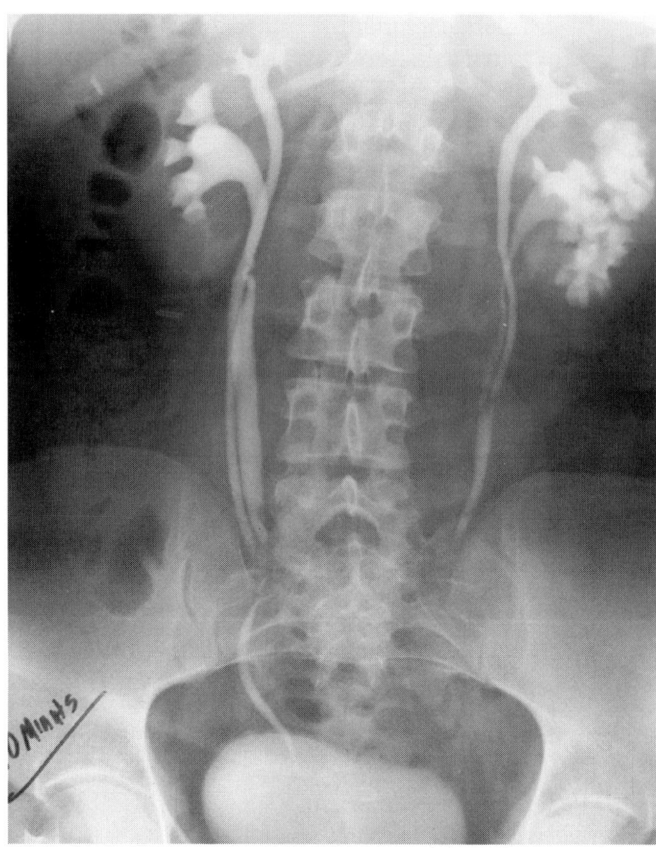

Figure 2–12. Congenital megacalycosis. There are bilateral duplications. Only the lower portion of the left kidney has the abnormal calyces. Distinction from reflux is important whenever this abnormality is suspected.

abnormality is due to an aperistalsis or adynamic distal segment of ureter that may be obstructing or nonobstructing. Dilatation may occur over a varying length. The dilated proximal segment has normal peristalsis. Clinically, these patients usually present in childhood. Males are more often affected, and the left kidney is affected more than the right. At urography, there will be dilatation of the ureter proximal to a segment of nondilated ureter. Severe cases may show complete dilatation of a ureter and dilatation of the renal pelvis and calyces. Atrophy of the kidney with significant delayed visualization at intravenous urography can also occur. Differentiation from a dilated but nonobstructed ureter is best performed with diuretic radionuclide studies. When the distal segment cannot be visualized, confirmation of primary obstructed megaureter can be obtained at retrograde pyelography. With ureterovesicular joint (UVJ) obstruction versus UPJ obstruction, dilatation of the proximal ureter observed by ultrasound may assist with the diagnosis.

CONGENITAL MEGACALYCOSIS

Congenital megacalycosis is a congenital anomaly in which there are enlarged calyces. Many of these patients have an increased number of calyces (more than 20) (Fig. 2–12). This diagnosis can be made only when there has not been prior obstruction and there is no evidence of reflux. Clinically these patients may present with infection or stone formation caused by stasis of urine in the enlarged calyces. However, the patients have a normal serum creatinine and creatinine clearance. This helps to distinguish this abnormality from either reflux or postobstructive atrophy. The condition is usually unilateral. At urography, contrast material reaches the abnormal calyx at the same time as it reaches calyces in the normal kidney, but the total opacification of the collecting system is delayed because of the increased volume of these dilated calyces. The proximal ureter and renal pelvis are usually normal in caliber. Diuretic renogra-

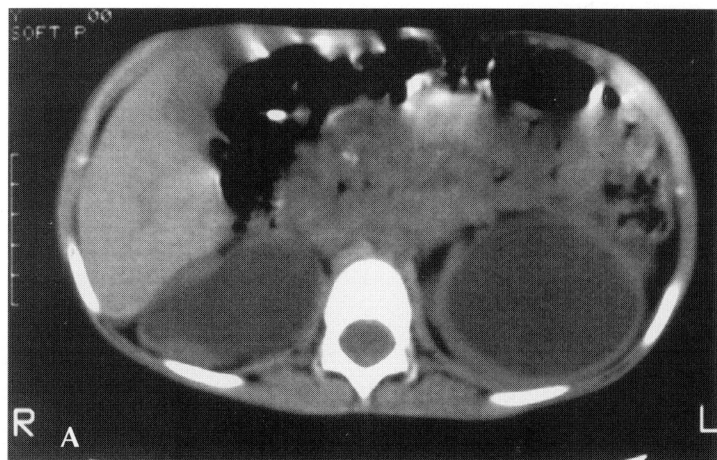

Figure 2.13. A. Bilateral hydronephrosis from Eagle–Barrett syndrome. B. Four images from a CT in the same patient show a dilated bladder and deficient abdominal wall musculature.

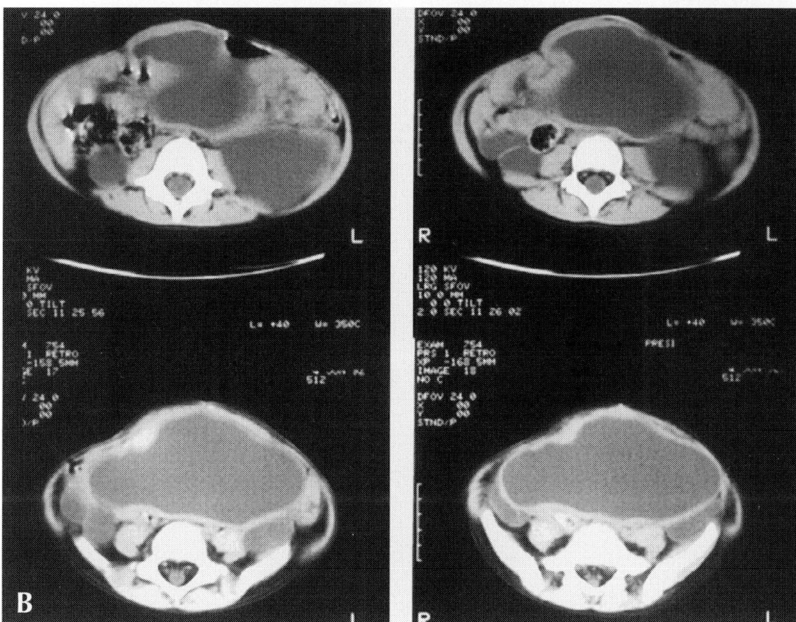

phy with technetium-99m DPTA is useful to differentiate this condition from urinary tract obstruction.

EAGLE–BARRETT SYNDROME OR PRUNE-BELLY SYNDROME

The Eagle–Barrett or prune-belly syndrome consists of the triad of absent or deficient abdominal wall musculature, cryptorchidism, and ureteric dilatation. In this syndrome, there is marked dilatation, elongation, and tortuosity of the ureters. This is true even though no obstruction is present. These patients usually have reflux. The muscle and fibrous tissue of the ureteric wall is abnormal. This leads to abnormal peristalsis. The same type of histologic findings may be found in the bladder, which is often dilated but nontrabeculated. These patients have a dilated prostatic urethra and a hypoplastic prostate with an absent to small verumontanum. A utricular diverticulum may also occur. The syndrome's effects range from near normal function with minimal symptoms to early death in the neonatal period. Renal dysplasia and hydronephrosis may be associated with pulmonary hypoplasia. Excretory urography and ultrasound will demonstrate the dilated collecting system (Fig. 2–13).

Chapter

3

Nephrocalcinosis and Nephrolithiasis

Stones visualized radiographically in the kidneys may be due to either nephrocalcinosis or nephrolithiasis. Nephrocalcinosis implies that there are calcium deposits within the substance of the kidney; stone densities located in the collecting system are referred to as nephrolithiasis. Table 3–1 summarizes the types of stones and their radiographic features.

NEPHROCALCINOSIS

Nephrocalcinosis is divided into cortical nephrocalcinosis and medullary nephrocalcinosis (Fig. 3–1). Corresponding to the distribution of calcification seen radiographically, cortical nephrocalcinosis occurs due to diseases that cause damage to cortical cells with resultant change in cellular pH, precipitation of calcium salts, and dystrophic calcification. Cortical necrosis due to ischemia or chronic glomerulonephritis is a common cause of this phenomenon.

Medullary nephrocalcinosis occurs in hypercalcemic states such as hyperparathyroidism, sarcoidosis, immobilization, hypervitaminosis D, milk alkalai syndrome, and neoplastic disorders. Distal renal tubular acidosis also causes medullary calcification. Medullary sponge kidney causes medullary calcification and is discussed in the next section.

Diffuse calcification of both kidneys involving both cortex and medulla is usually due to increased oxylates. Diffuse nephrocalcinosis occurs when oxalate levels are high, as with ethylene glycol poisoning, methoxyflurane anesthesia, or increased absorption of oxalates with inflammatory bowel disease. Unilateral diffuse calcification should raise suspicion for tuberculosis.

Detecting Nephrolithiasis and Nephrocalcinosis

Proper radiographic technique must be used to detect stones in the kidneys. Scattered radiation, which degrades the image, can be prevented by collimating the x ray to the kidney as tightly as possible. Nephrolithiasis occurs for many different types of stones (Table 3–1). Many of these stones can be detected by plain x rays if proper technique is used, which means using low kilovolts peak (kVp). However, 30 to 50 percent of stones are difficult to see on plain film. Stones, such as uric acid stones, that cannot be visualized on plain film are termed radi-

TABLE 3–1. **Types of Stones and Their Radiologic Features**

Types of Stones	Percentage of Stones	Opacity	Comments
Calcium oxylate	34	Very opaque	
Calcium oxylate plus calcium phosphate	34	Very opaque	Occasionally associated with infection.
Calcium phosphate	6	Very opaque	Occasionally associated with infection. Form in alkaline urine.
Magnesium ammonium phosphate often mixed with calcium phosphate	15	Intermediate (the more calcium, the more opaque)	Frequently associated with infection *(Proteus mirabilis).* Form with urine pH >7.2. 70 percent of staghorns.
Uric acid	7	Lucent	50 percent of these are in patients with gout. Form in acid urine.
Cystine	3	Lucent	Form in acid urine.
Matrix	less than 1	Lucent	Microproteins/mucopoly-saccharide associated with infection.
Xanthine	rare	Lucent	

olucent. Tomograms will be more sensitive than plain films because they help to avoid some of the problems with overlying stool and bowel gas. The most sensitive way to detect a stone is by using CT. While ultrasound is probably the most sensitive method of detecting hydronephrosis, abdominal CT is more sensitive for the actual detection of the stone. If a CT scan is used to search for a renal stone, it should be performed without IV contrast. Intravenous contrast will obscure the stone because the contrast will be excreted by the collecting system. Even a stone that is radiolucent when using plain x rays may be seen on CT because of higher contrast.

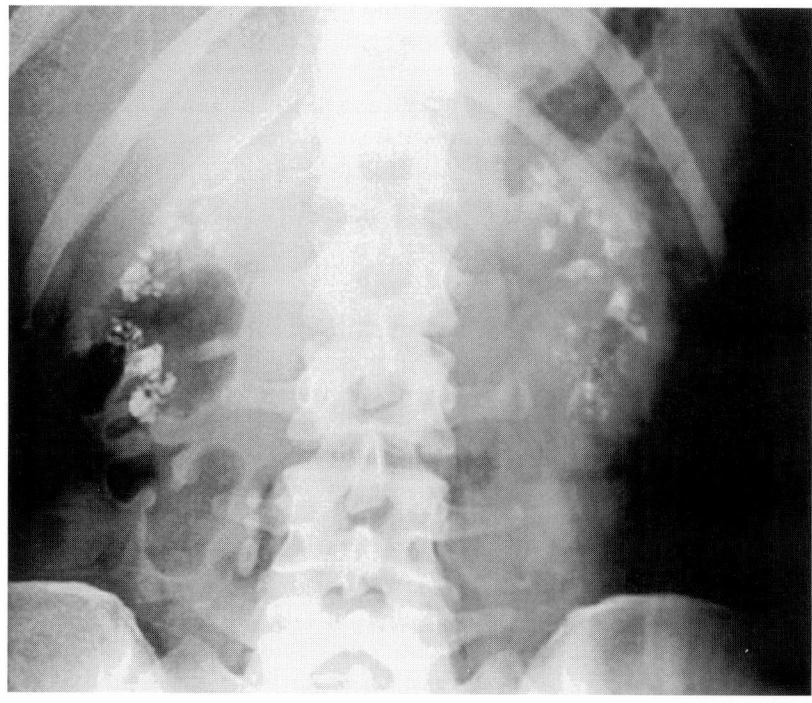

Figure 3–1. Medullary nephrocalcinosis and nephrolithiasis.

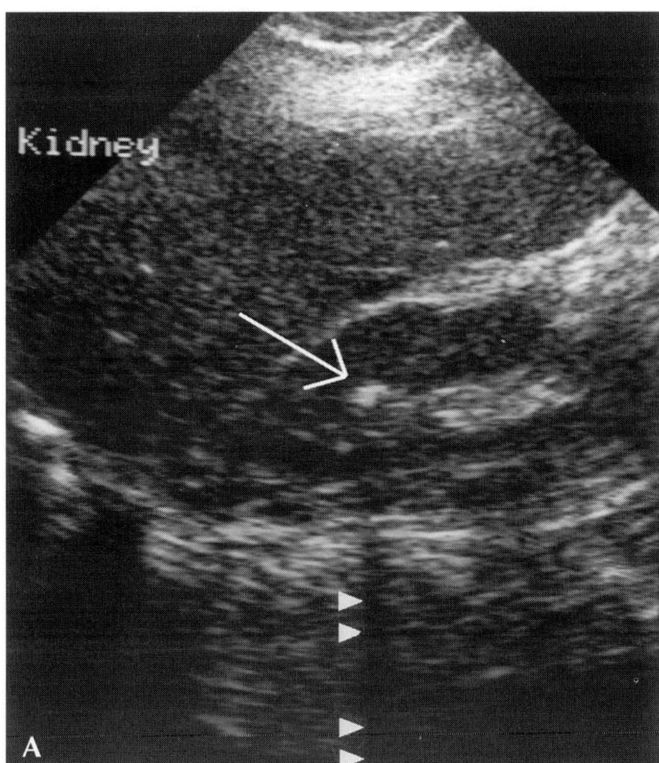

Figure 3–2. A. A stone (arrow) in the upper pole of the right kidney with a shadow (arrowheads). **B.** Echogenic renal sinus fat (F), making the echogenic focus less obvious. A shadow (arrow) helps to identify the stone.

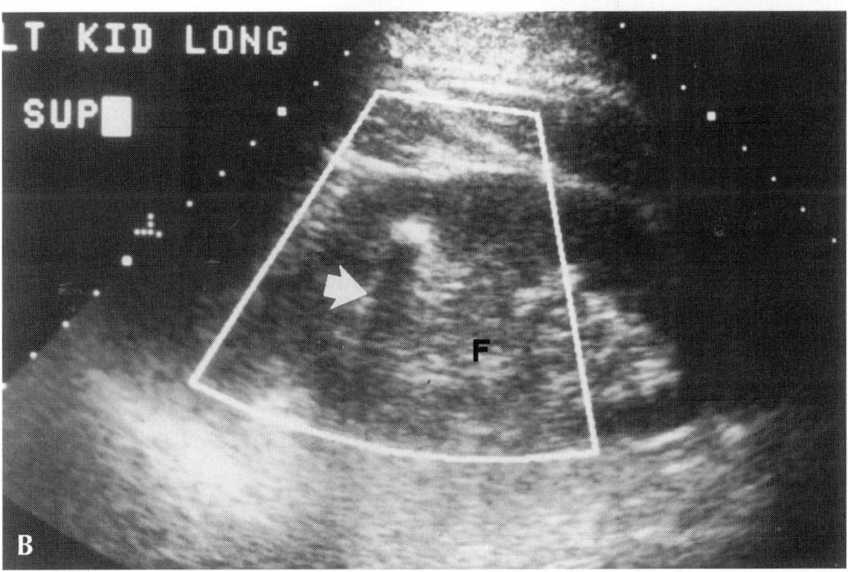

Ultrasound is frequently used to search for stones. Estimates of the sensitivity of ultrasound have ranged from 60 percent to 90 percent. The ultrasound findings of stone disease are a bright echogenic reflector with a shadow behind it (Fig. 3–2*A*). The echogenic reflector may be obscured by echogenic fat in the renal sinus (Fig. 3–2*B*). Also, if the stone is not within the focal zone of the transducer, it may not be visualized. If an echogenic focus without shadowing is identified, the diagnosis of stone is uncertain. Using transducers with a higher frequency and superior resolution may help to produce a shadow and confirm that a stone or calcification is present.

Calcium Stones

Calcium stones are the easiest to see radiographically and account for about 90 percent of the stone disease in the United States. The majority of these stones are calcium oxylate. Almost 50 percent of calcium oxalate stones are associated with hypercalciuria in the absence of hypercalcemia. This condition is known as idiopathic hypercalciuria. Idiopathic hypercalciuria may be due to either increased intestinal absorption of calcium, known as absorptive hypercalciuria, or a renal leak of calcium. Resorptive hypercalciuria occurs but is synonymous with hyperparathyroidism in that bone resorption and intestinal absorption of calcium are increased and there is usually hypercalcemia. Calcium oxalate stones are also found in patients with hypercalcemia (e.g., hyperparathyroidism, sarcoidosis, or malignancy), hyperuricosuria, hypocitraturia, and hyperoxaluria.

Hyperoxaluria as a cause of calcium oxalate stone disease may occur in a primary form due to congenital hyperoxaluria. The secondary form of hyperoxaluria occurs with intestinal conditions such as malabsorption, steatorrhea, intestinal bypass surgery, blind loop syndrome, and hyperperistalsis. These conditions lead to excessive absorption of oxalate because calcium is not available in the bowel to bind with the oxalate. The other type of calcium stone disease, accounting for 10 percent of nephroliths, is due to calcium phosphate stones. These often occur with hypercalcemia from causes such as primary hyperparathroidism, prolonged immobilization, sarcoidosis, hypervitaminosis D, milk alkalai syndrome, and widespread metastatic disease to bone. Many stones have a mixed composition.

Struvite Stones and Steghorn Calculi

Chronic urinary tract infections are associated with struvite or magnesium ammonium phosphate stones. The classic infecting organism is *Proteus mirabilis,* which contains the enzyme urease. Urease cleaves urea into ammonia and ammonium. The infected urine becomes alkaline, producing a supersatured solution of magnesium ammonium phosphate. Magnesium ammonium phosphate stones form when the urine pH is above 7.2. These stones grow rapidly and frequently produce staghorn calculi, which give a radiographic cast to the collecting system or a portion of it (Fig. 3–3). The radiographic density of these stones is determined by the amount of calcium. Pure magnesium ammonium stones are only faintly visible. The radiographic appearance of a staghorn calculus is easily recognized. The calculus itself may be obscured by contrast. On noncontrasted CT, a large dense structure will be seen occupying much of the renal pelvis.

Uric Acid Stones

In some patients an increased concentration of free uric acid will occur. Uric acid stones may occur in this situation. Predisposition to the formation of these stones may occur in patients who take medications that acidify the urine. Patients who have chronic diarrhea or an ileostomy causing aciduria may also form uric acid stones. Patients with hyperuricemia are also prone to form uric acid stones. However, only 25 percent of patients with gout form stones. Some drugs such as aspirin or thiazide diuretics may cause increased excretion of uric acid and predispose patients to the formation of uric acid stones. Neoplastic disease with high levels of purine metabolism such as multiple myeloma or leukemia may also produce uric acid stones. Uric acid stones are radiolucent and are poorly seen on an abdominal radiograph (Fig. 3–4). However, they are well seen on a CT scan.

Cystine Stones

These stones occur in patients who have cystinuria. These patients have a defect in the tubular reabsorption of the amino acids cystine, ornathine, lysine, and arginine (COLA). This is an autosomal recessive trait. An excess of cystine in the urine leads to the precipitation of stones. Usually, the only clinical manifestation is the formation of renal stones. Cystine stones may occur as early as the teenage years. Cystine stones are relatively radiolucent. This means that on plain film the stones may be

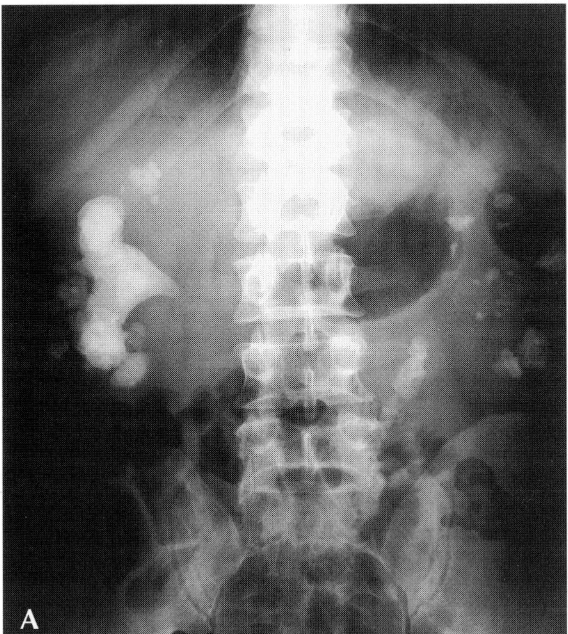

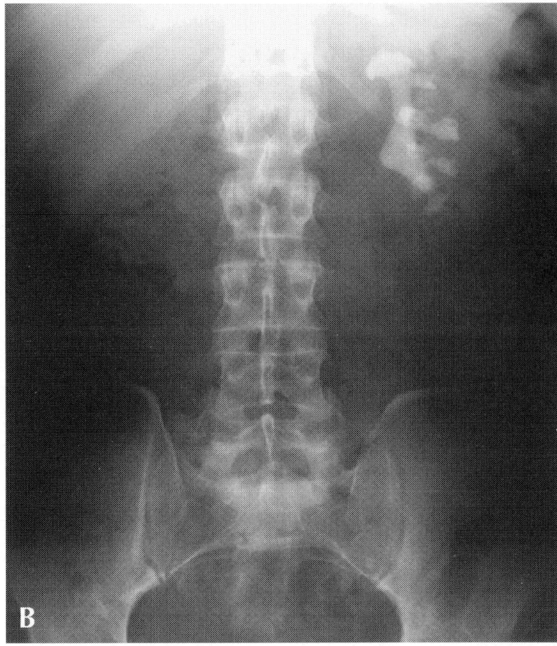

Figure 3–3. A. A right staghorn calculus with other areas of nephrocalcinosis. **B.** A different patient with a left staghorn calculus. These are magnesium ammonium phosphate stones.

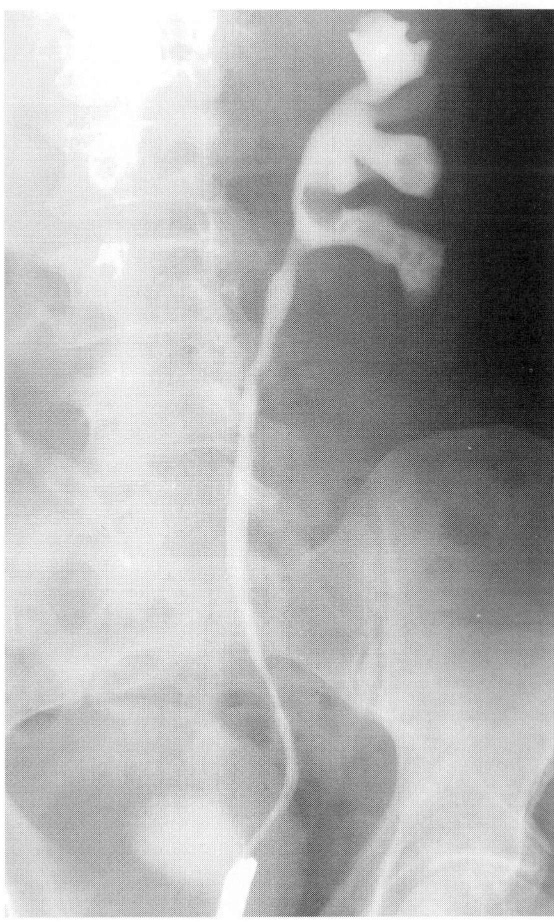

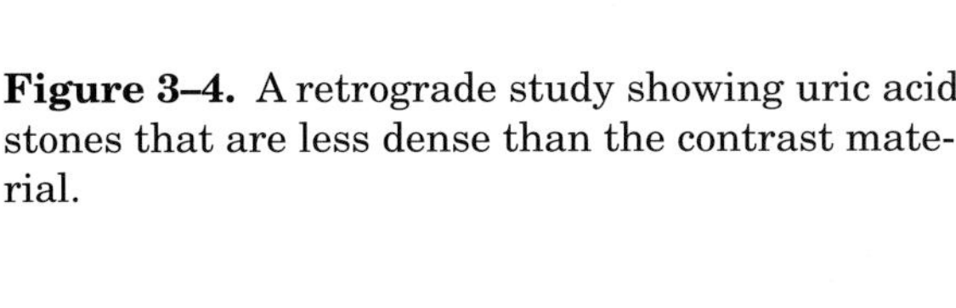

Figure 3–4. A retrograde study showing uric acid stones that are less dense than the contrast material.

faintly visible, but on contrasted studies the stones appear lucent because the contrast is more dense. Some cystine stones may contain calcium and therefore will be visible as a stone on a plain, noncontrasted radiograph. A CT scan may still detect them, as will ultrasound.

Hydrocalyx with Milk of Calcium

At times, a fluid calcium layer may be seen in either a diverticulum or a hydrocalyx of the kidney. This is known as "milk of calcium" and is usually found in the upper pole of the kidney. Milk of calcium consists of a colloidal suspension of calcific granules. If the patient is supine and a plain film is obtained, the fluid calcium layer cannot be appreciated and appears as a poorly defined density. When an upright film or a CT scan is obtained, the fluid calcium layer may be seen.

Obstructions Secondary to a Stone

Obstructions secondary to a stone occur when a stone passes through the renal pelvis into the ureter and obstructs, most commonly at the ureteropelvic junction, the pelvic brim, or the ureterovesical junction (Fig. 3–5). The ureterovesical junction is the most common site for obstruction. After acute obstruction has occurred, renal blood flow decreases, ureteral pressure increases, and ultimately there is a decrease in the glomerular filtration rate. Radiographically, the obstructed kidney appears enlarged. After injection of contrast material, there is a decrease in the amount of enhancement when compared to the normal side. However, as time passes, the nephrogram becomes progressively more intense on the obstructed side. There may be a striated appearance secondary to contrast material retained in the collecting ducts. At times, the contrast

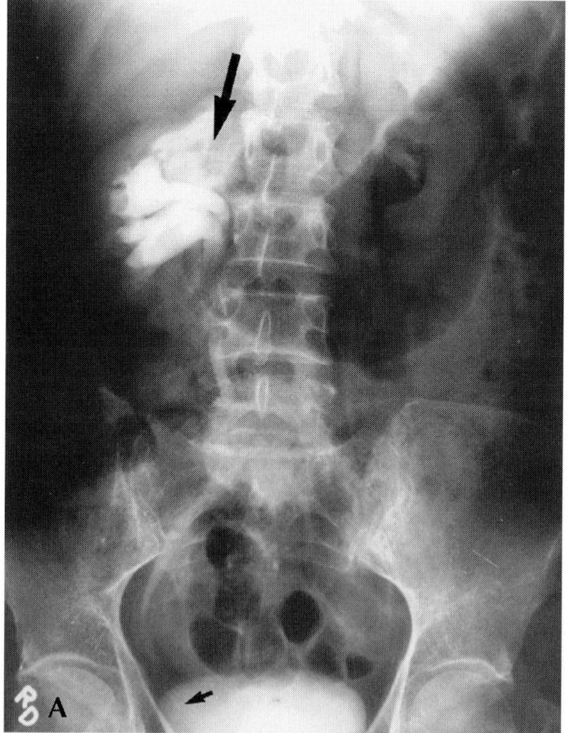

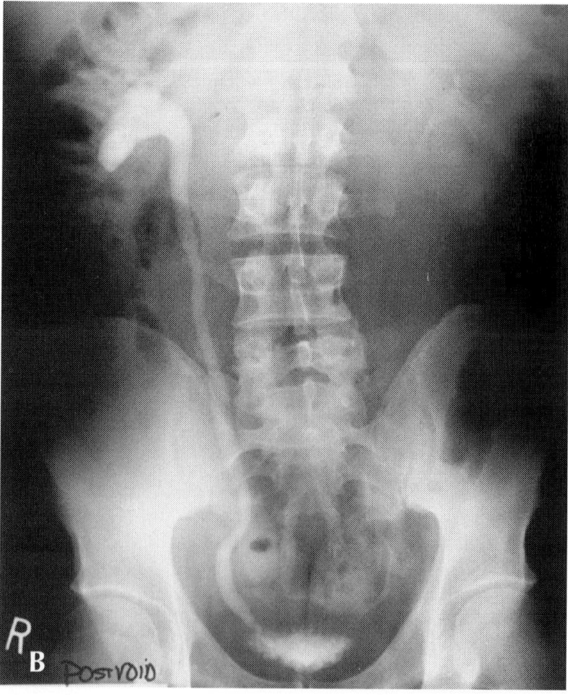

Figure 3–5. A. The stone at the right ureterovesical junction (small arrow) cannot be definitely identified. However, the dilated ureter indicates obstruction. The obstruction is high grade and causes pyelosinus backflow (large arrow). **B.** A different patient with hydroureter due to a stone at the ureterovesical junction. The surrounding contrast obscures the stone.

material may not appear in the collecting system until 24 hours after injection. The intensity of the nephrogram does not correlate with the duration of obstruction. After a number of days have gone by, renal function may be diminished so that only a very faint nephrogram will be seen. Intravenous urography is more sensitive than ultrasonography for acute obstruction because in early obstruction, dilatation of the calyces and pelvis may not develop for a number of hours and in some patients may not develop at all. The diuresis produced by the volume of contrast material may also help detect obstruction. The diuresis induced by high-osmolality contrast material may even cause an acute obstructing stone to pass during the course of the study. The patient usually reports that the pain has resolved suddenly. The previously obstructed system may return to normal quickly.

The earliest radiographic sign of obstruction and hydronephrosis seen on intravenous urography is blunting of the forniceal angles. Alternating radiolucent and radiopaque stripes in the kidney are felt to represent contrast material in dilated tubules and collecting ducts in the medullary rays. Another sign, called the calyceal "crescent sign," represents contrast material in collecting ducts.

Intravenous urography (IVU) is quite accurate at detecting ureteral obstruction. It also provides physiologic information and can detect anatomic anomalies and abnormalities. Disadvantages are that the test requires intravenous contrast administration, can take hours if it is positive, and when negative provides no information about other possible causes of flank pain. Intravenous urography depends on plain films (with their low sensitivity) to detect, localize, and size stones.

Spiral CT without intravenous contrast has recently come into widespread use. It has approximately a 95 percent sensitivity, 98 percent specificity, and 97 percent accuracy for diagnosis of ureteral stone disease. A volume of data is collected from the top of the kidneys (about T11) to the pubic symphysis using 5-mm collimation. This technique allows accurate stone localization that is important if ESWL (Extracorporeal Shock Wave Lithotripsy), ureteroscopy, or stone retrieval are planned. In addition to visualization of the stone in the ureter, other helpful signs include ureteral dilatation, soft tissue stranding in the perinephric fat (Fig. 3–6*A*), dilatation of the intrarenal collecting system, and renal enlargement (Fig. 3–6*A*). The presence of unilateral ureteral dilatation plus perinephric stranding has a positive predictive value of 96 percent; absence of both signs has a negative predictive value of 93 percent. Problems with spiral CT include phleboliths near the ureter that may simulate stones. In addition, the study gives no functional information, which may be important for treatment planning. Eighty percent of ureteral stones will have a "rim sign" that consists of thickening and irregularity of the ureteric wall around a stone (Fig. 3–6*B*). This "rim sign" is present more often with stones less than 4 mm in size.

About 30 percent of patients with flank pain will have a cause other than stone disease, and CT is quite helpful for diagnosing these other diseases, including appendicitis, diverticular disease, and adnexal disease.

Medullary Sponge Kidney

Patients with medullary sponge kidney have dilated collecting ducts. These ectatic ducts may either be cystic or cylindrical in shape and cause an increase in the size of the papilla. The calyx increases in diameter and has a flattened appearance. The kidney may sometimes be increased in size. Small calcifications in the region of the papillae can sometimes be seen. These patients have a normal life expectancy and are often free of any urinary tract symptoms. They do have a propensity to form stones (Fig. 3–7).

Radiographically, plain films demonstrate medullary nephrocalcinosis, but often there are no findings. After the injection of intravenous contrast material, contrast material may be seen extending from the calyx into the papillae in a linear fashion. This contrast material outlines the enlarged collecting duct and has been described as resembling a paintbrush (Fig. 3–8). These linear striations in the papillae are suggestive of a diagnosis. The demonstration of nephrocalcinosis is further evidence sup-

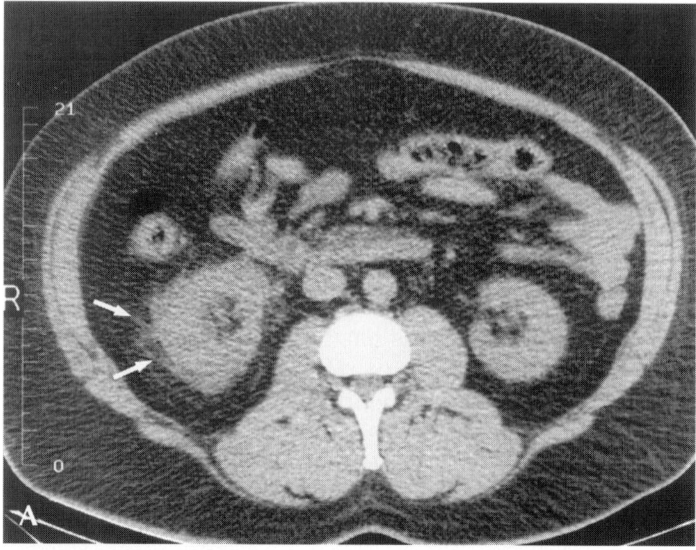

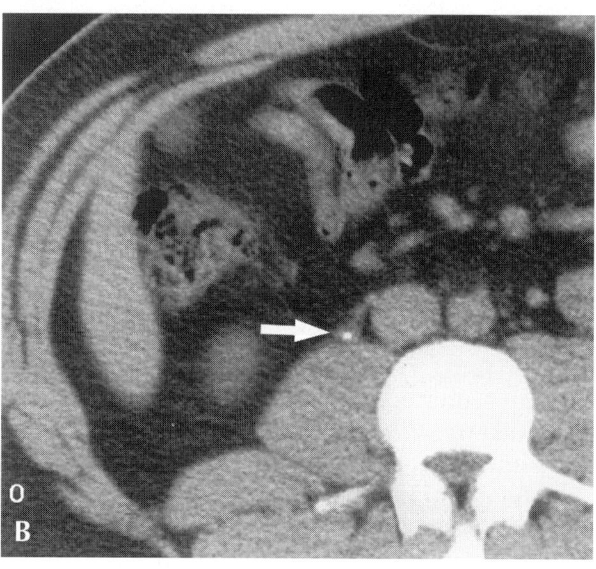

Figure 3–6. A. This noncontrast CT scan shows s swollen right kidney with stranding (arrows) due to an obstructed ureter. **B.** A CT scan showing a stone (arrow) in midureter with the soft tissue rim sign.

porting the diagnosis. Computed tomography is better at detecting the nephrocalcinosis. Calcifications in the region of the medullary pyramids in a pattern of rings have been described on CT. At ultrasound, increased echogenicity secondary to the nephrocalcinosis may be seen in the region of the medullary pyramids. If only small amounts of calcification are present, there may not be shadowing. Medullary sponge kidney is one cause of medullary calcifications that may lead to calcifications occurring in only one kidney or a portion of one kidney. Most other causes of medullary calcification are bilateral and symmetric.

Phleboliths

Phleboliths may be confused with urinary tract stones. This is especially true in the pelvis. Phleboliths are typically rounded with a central area of lucency (Fig. 3–9). They are often more caudal than the distal ureter. After contrast is injected, they may sometimes be shown to be outside of the bladder or the path of the ureters. Old films may be helpful to ensure that the calcification has been present for a long period of time, suggesting that it is a phlebolith. The term *phlebolith* means "vein stone." These are generally felt to occur as a result of thrombosis of

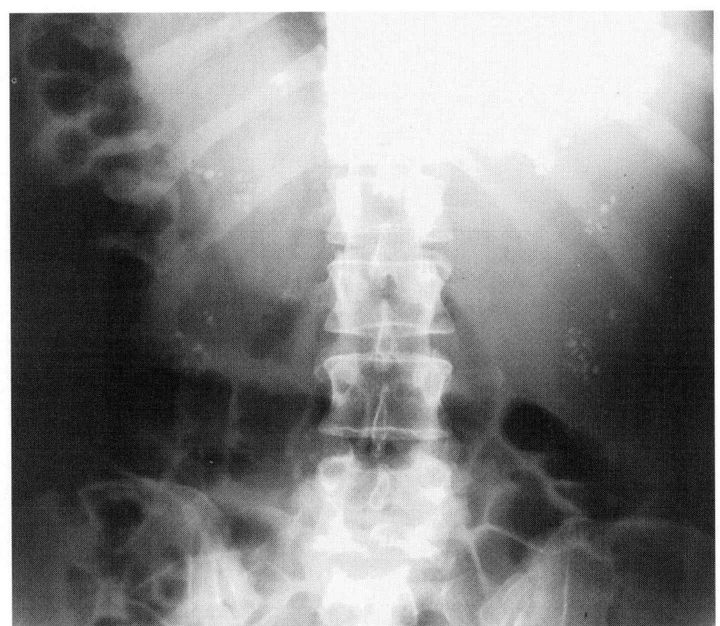

Figure 3–7. Stones due to medullary sponge kidney.

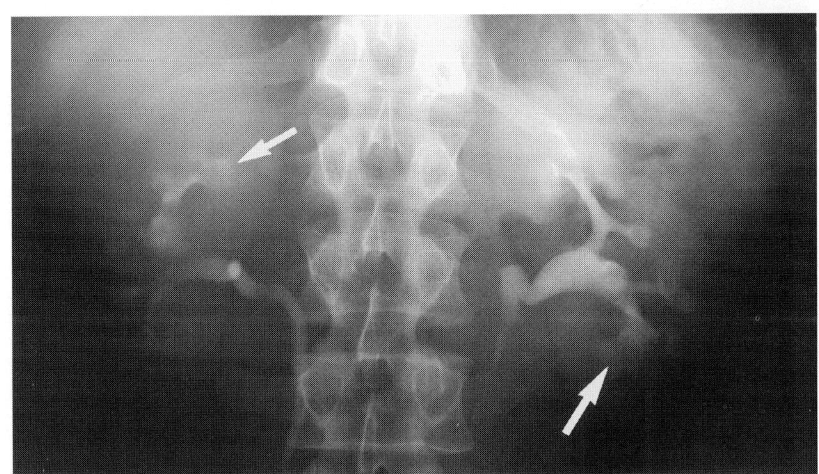

Figure 3–8. These striations in the papillae resemble a paintbrush (arrows). This appearance is typical of medullary sponge kidney after contrast.

the pelvic veins. It may not be possible to distinguish a phlebolith from a stone with a high degree of certainty without injecting contrast.

Renal Tubular Acidosis/Hyperparathyroidism/Nephrocalcinosis

Patients who have distal renal tubular acidosis (RTA) are unable to form an acid urine because of an inability to secrete hydrogen against a concentration gradient (Type I). In the complete form of renal tubular acidosis, patients have non-anion gap metabolic acidosis, hyperchloremia, hypokalemia, hypercalciuria, and a urine pH consistently above 6.0. There is also an incomplete form of renal tubular acidosis in which the serum electrolytes remain normal, but calcium is insoluble in the urine because of lack of citrate. Both of these types of renal tubular acidosis are known as distal renal tubular acidosis. Patients with distal renal tubular acidosis have problems with muscle weakness and rickets and osteomalacia (Fig. 3–10*A*). Children may become growth retarded. About three-quarters of the patients with the distal form of renal tubu-

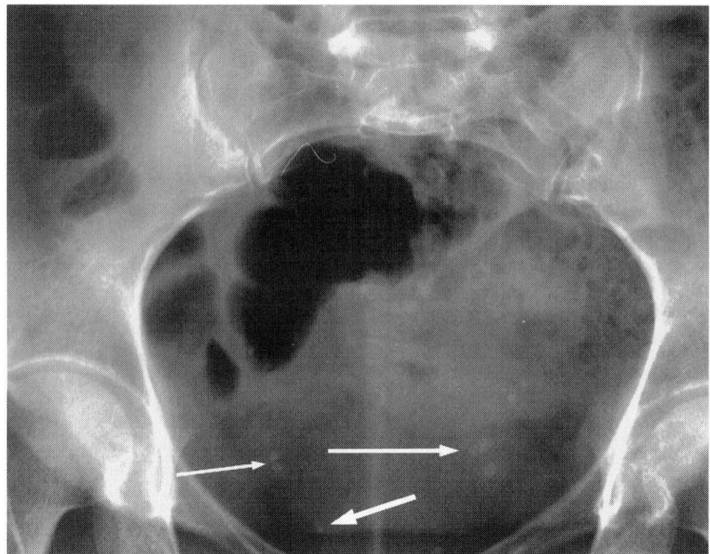

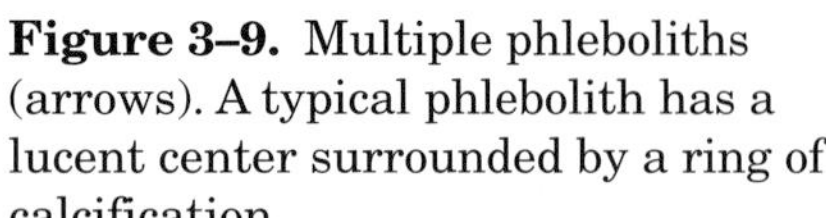

Figure 3–9. Multiple phleboliths (arrows). A typical phlebolith has a lucent center surrounded by a ring of calcification.

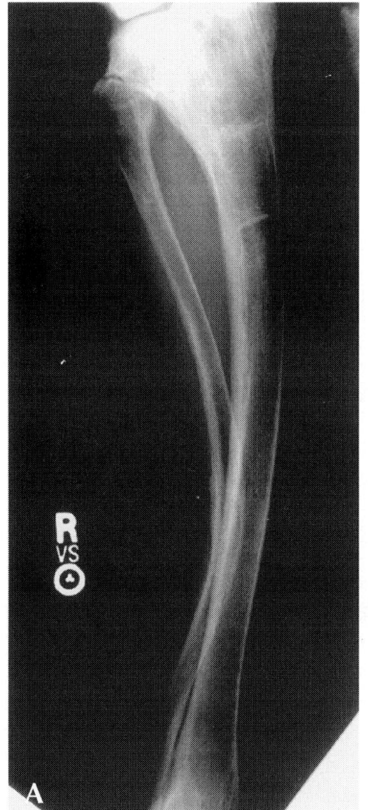

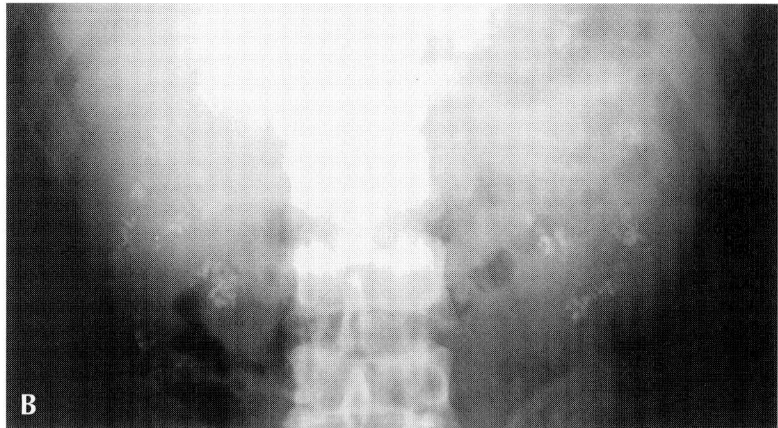

Figure 3–10. A. Renal osteodystrophy secondary to renal failure from renal tubular acidosis. **B.** Medullary nephrocalcinosis from renal tubular acidosis in the same patient.

lar acidosis have medullary nephrocalcinosis and nephrolithiasis (Fig. 3–10*B*). A second form of RTA occurs due to impaired absorption of bicarbonate in the proximal tubule (Type II). Stone formation does not occur in the proximal form of renal tubular acidosis because citrate excretion is increased.

Primary hyperparathyroidism occurs when the patient has an adenoma, a carcinoma, or hyperplasia of the parathyroid gland. This results in excess secretion of parathyroid hormone. These patients have an increased propensity to form calcium oxalate or calcium phosphate renal stones. Radiographically, hyperparathyroidism causes medullary nephrocalcinosis.

Chapter

4

Upper Tract Tumors

RENAL CELL CARCINOMA

A renal mass may be an incidental finding on ultrasound, computed tomography (CT), or intravenous urography. It may also be revealed as a result of a workup for hematuria. Anytime a solid renal mass is detected, there is a significant risk of renal cell carcinoma. While renal cell carcinomas usually occur in patients over 40 years of age, they may occur in children and in patients in their 20s. There is a male to female ratio of about 3:1.

Renal cell carcinomas are felt to arise from proximal tubular cells. Between 80 and 95 percent of renal cell carcinomas are hypervascular, and a minority are hypovascular. Some risk factors for renal cell carcinoma include tobacco use, phenacetin, obesity, the autosomal recessive disorder of Von Hippel-Lindau syndrome, and acquired renal cystic disease seen in patients undergoing dialysis.

On intravenous urography (IVU), renal cell carcinomas usually present as a localized bulge or contour abnormality, especially during the nephrogram phase of the study. If the tumor is located in the central part of the kidney, there may be no detectable abnormality, although even centrally located tumors may cause displacement or obliteration of the renal pelvis, infundibula, or calyces (Fig. 4–1*A*,*B*). An increase in the distance between a calyx and the outer margin of the cortex may be a less direct indicator of neoplastic disease. Adenocarcinomas usually enhance after intravenous contrast but do not retain the contrast material. Therefore, they are less dense than surrounding normal kidney.

Overall, the sensitivity of IVU for adenocarcinoma is about 70 percent. Computed tomography has an estimated sensitivity of 90 percent because visualization of those tumors that do not produce a contour abnormality is possible. Computed tomography also offers the added benefit of more precise staging. Because 80 to 90 percent of adenocarcinomas are hypervascular, these tumors may blush, especially if scanned during an arterial phase. However, if it is scanned during the tubular phase or after a 90-second delay, the tumor may appear less dense than surrounding normal tissue (Fig. 4–2). Appropriate technique for the evaluation of a renal mass by CT scan is essential. Technical points include the use of nonenhanced and enhanced images to look for evidence of differential contrast enhancement in the tumor, thin cuts (5 mm or 3 mm) through the parenchyma, and bolus contrast infusion

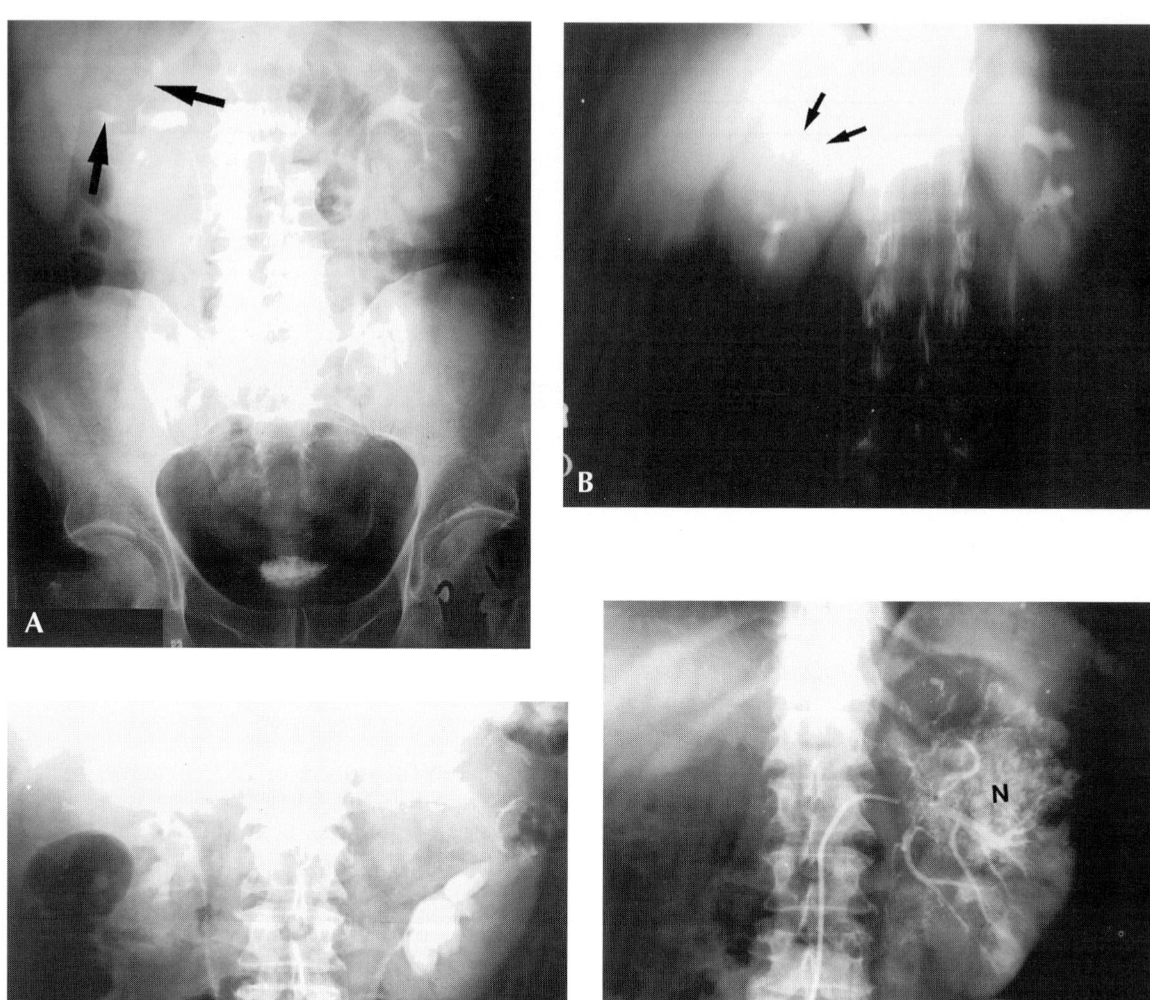

Figure 4–1. A. In the upper pole the calyces (arrows) are spread secondary to a renal cell carcinoma. **B.** A different patient shows bowing and stretching of the upper-pole calyx (arrows). **C.** The mass in the upper pole of the left kidney is pushing the left collecting system down. **D.** This angiogram of the patient in **C** shows the extent of the tumor. There is widespread neovascularity (N).

with proper timing. A benign lesion should enhance by no more than 15 Hounsfield units (H) (Fig. 4–3). However, some authorities use 10 H, others use 20 H.

Magnetic resonance imaging without gadolinium will detect only about 63 percent of small renal tumors because the cancer often has signal characteristics similar to those of normal kidneys. Gadolinium greatly improves this sensitivity. After gadolinium, a mass should not increase in signal (i.e., enhance). If it does, then renal cell carcinoma should be suspected. The usual renal cell carcinoma is hypoechoic on ultrasound (Fig. 4–4) when compared to adjacent normal renal parenchyma. However, many renal cell carcinomas are difficult to see on ultrasound because there is very little difference between the appearance of the cancer and adjacent kidney. It is

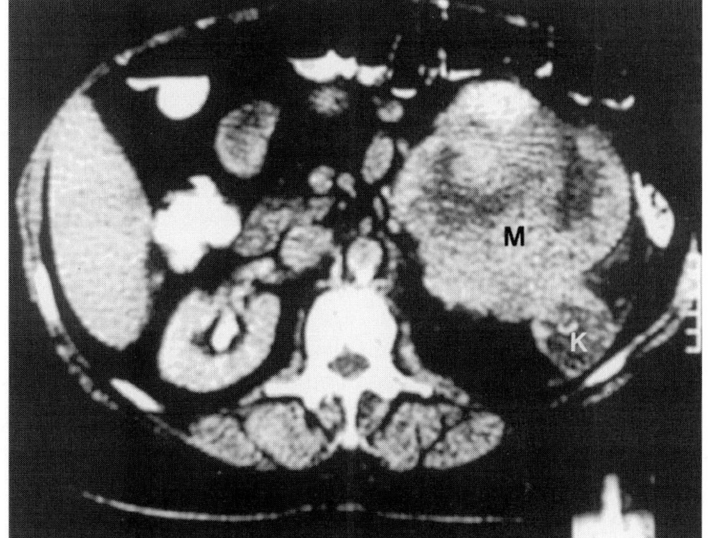

Figure 4–2. A large mass (M) projects anteriorly from an atrophic left kidney (K). Most of this mass enhances less than the cortex of the right kidney. This is common for a renal cell carcinoma.

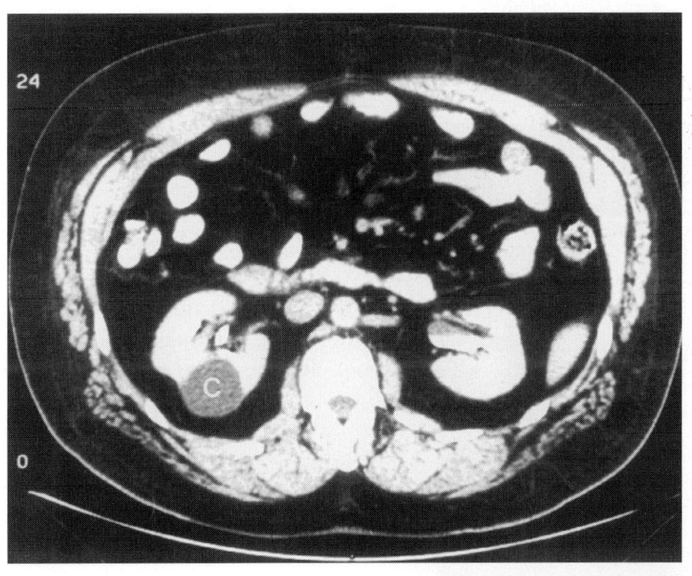

Figure 4–3. Postcontrast images of a simple cyst (C). Lesions such as this should have Hounsfield units (H) measured before and after contrast. More than 15 H of enhancement suggests a renal cell carcinoma. This lesion showed approximately 10 H of enhancement.

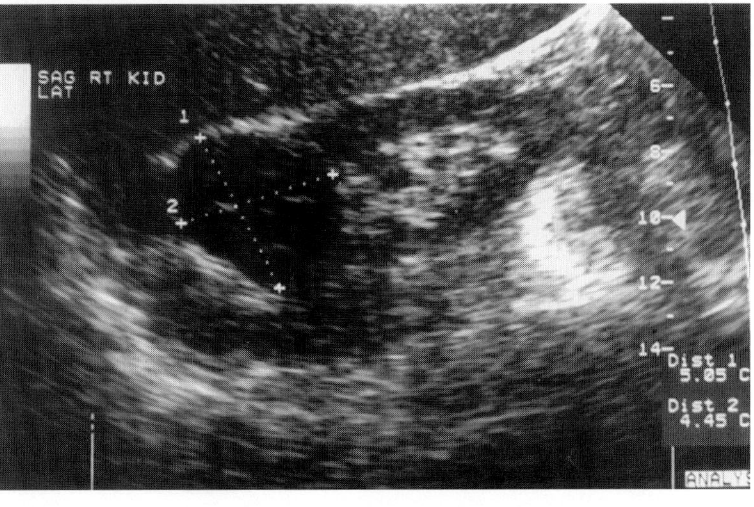

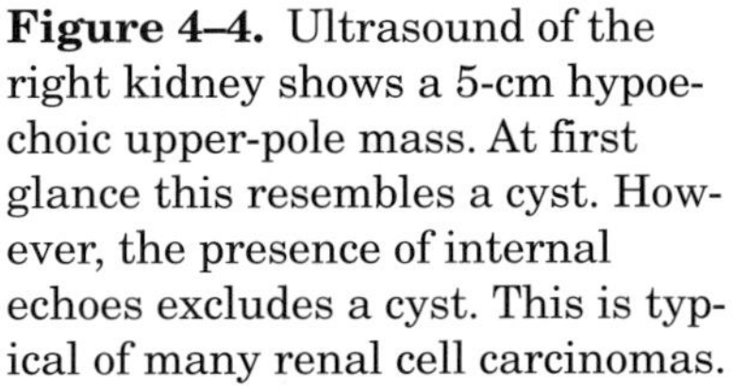
Figure 4–4. Ultrasound of the right kidney shows a 5-cm hypoechoic upper-pole mass. At first glance this resembles a cyst. However, the presence of internal echoes excludes a cyst. This is typical of many renal cell carcinomas.

estimated that ultrasound is only about 70 percent sensitive for the detection of renal cell carcinomas.

The Robson staging of renal cell carcinoma is as follows:

I. Tumor confined to the kidney.
II. Tumor spread to perinephric fat but within Gerota's fascia.
III. Tumor with
   A. Renal vein and/or IVC (Inferior Vena Cava) invasion.
   B. Regional node metastases.
   C. Venous invasion and lymph node invasion.
IV. Tumor with
   A. Extension through renal fascia to adjacent organs.
   B. Distant metastases.

Both CT and MRI are used in the staging process to determine if a tumor is confined to the kidney or confined within Gerota's fascia. Renal vein invasion may be suspected if an enlarged expanded renal vein or IVC is seen, especially if these vessels do not enhance after contrast (Fig. 4–5). MRI may be more useful in detecting tumor clots in the IVC and right atrium (Fig. 4–6). We perform cardiac-gated MRI in the sagittal and axial planes. If a tumor clot is detected in the IVC, the differential diagnosis includes renal cell carcinoma, Wilm's tumor, adrenocortical carcinoma, and transitional cell carcinoma. Transesophageal echocardiography has also been used to evaluate the inferior vena cava for tumor clot. In the past, contrast venography was used, but this technique has largely been abandoned. When examining the IVC by contrasted CT, one should not mistake a mixing of contrast material and blood for tumor clot in the IVC. This mixing occurs where contrast material-

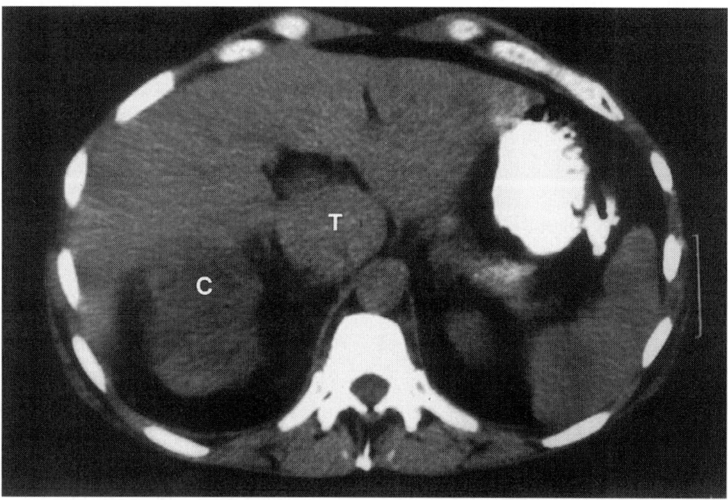

Figure 4–5. This noncontrasted CT shows a huge expanded IVC from a tumor clot (T). Renal cell carcinoma (C) is seen in the upper pole of the right kidney.

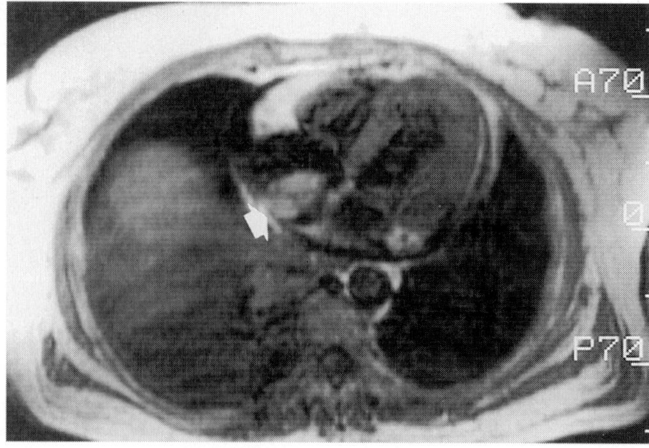

Figure 4–6. These MRI axial images of the heart show a tumor clot in the right atrium (arrow) from renal cell carcinoma.

enhanced blood from the renal vein drains into the IVC and swirls and mixes with nonenhanced blood from the IVC. The appearance can closely simulate a tumor clot.

In the past, angiography has been used in the evaluation of renal masses because up to 90 percent of renal cell carcinomas have neovascularity, that is, vessels that are disordered and do not conform to normal vascular patterns (Figs. 4–1*D,* 4–7). These vessels frequently lack a capillary bed and normal arterioles so that arteriovenous shunting may occur. Unfortunately, some renal cell carcinomas do not have this feature and other lesions such as renal abscesses may have abnormal vessels simulating neovascularity. Therefore, this technique has been supplanted by other imaging methods.

Calcification in a Renal Mass on Plain Films

An old saying ascribed to the evaluation of renal masses is "calcification means cancer" (Fig. 4–8). Typically, calcification in renal cell carcinoma is centrally located and nonlinear in nature. It is sometimes described as being amorphous. It may also be mottled or punctate. Renal cysts may also, at times, have calcifications. The calcification in a renal cyst

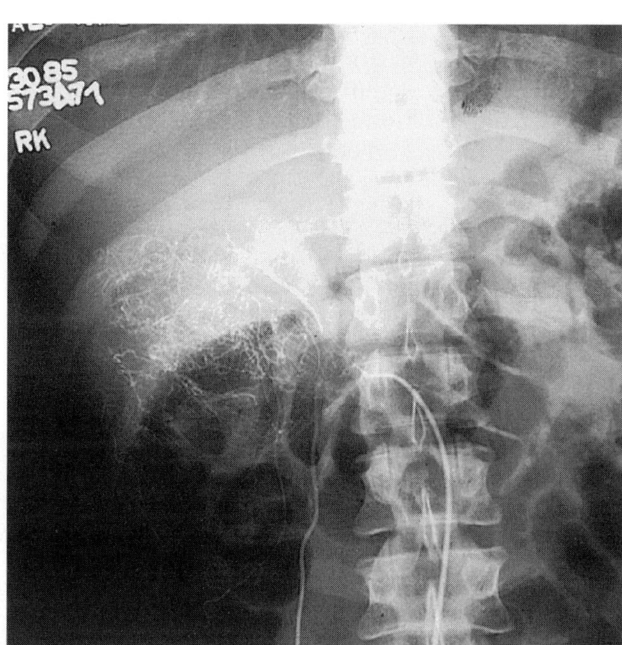

Figure 4–7. This angiogram of the right kidney shows extensive numbers of abnormal vessels in the upper pole in this renal cell carcinoma.

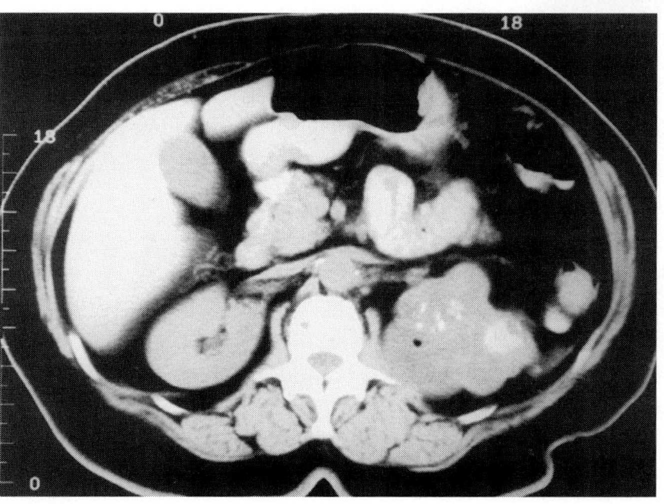

Figure 4–8. An irregular mass left kidney that is hypodense compared to a normal right kidney after contrast. This renal cell carcinoma has associated calcifications.

is usually peripheral, eggshell-thin, and linear. Calcification in a renal cell carcinoma occurs because of necrosis and dystrophic calcification. Of those masses that contain calcium in a nonperipheral location, about 90 percent are carcinoma. About 10 percent of adenocarcinomas have detectable calcium by plain film. By CT, this number increases to about 30 percent. Unfortunately, a small percentage of renal cell carcinomas will have peripheral linear calcification. Therefore, the pattern of calcification cannot be used with certainty to determine whether or not a lesion is likely to be malignant or benign. Calcification can be used with other evidence that may be available, which may include ureteral notching (reflecting collateral vessels) or tumor clot in the main renal vein. Tortuous densities after the administration of contrast may sometimes be identified in the fat around a kidney. These reflect dilated capsular arteries and veins.

Renal Cysts

A significant problem when evaluating kidneys is distinguishing between adenocarcinoma of the kidney and a benign renal cyst. In general, a renal cyst should be regular in shape, smooth, have thin, regular walls, and have a density that approximates water. There should be little or no change in the CT density between the nonenhanced and enhanced images (Fig. 4–3). On nonenhanced images the density should be between 0 and 20 H. Small lesions (less than 1.5 cm) are often a problem because volume averaging may lead to a falsely elevated Hounsfield measurement and the walls and contours may be difficult to evaluate.

Bosniak has devised a method of classifying renal cysts as to their malignant potential. Category I lesions are clearly simple cysts. Category II lesions also have little malignant potential. They may be minimally complex at CT, with thin smooth septa and/or smooth plaques of fine linear calcification in the wall. High-density cysts, usually from prior hemorrhage and measuring 10–100, also are in Category II (Fig. 4–9). On MRI a cyst that contains blood should have a high signal on both T1- and T2-weighted images.

Category III lesions have thick septa with

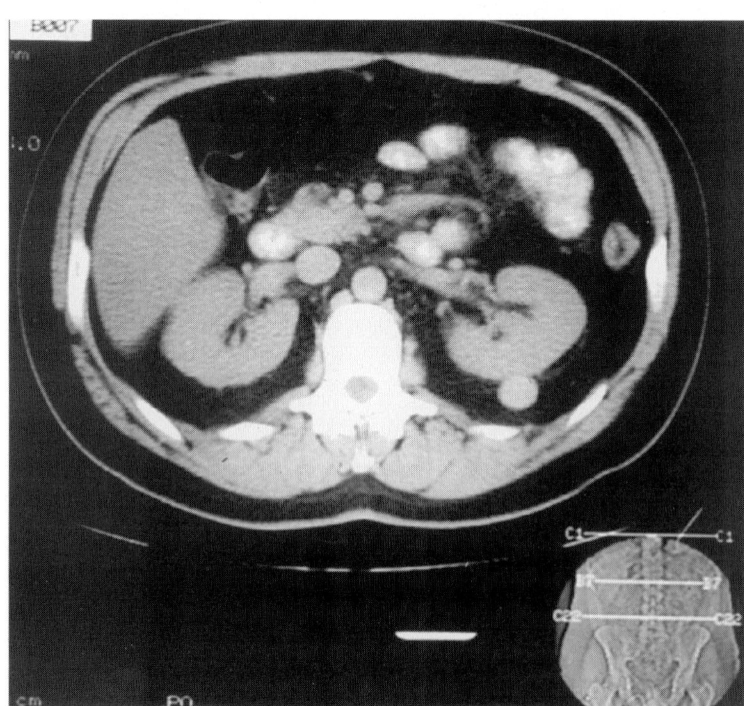

Figure 4–9. A 1-cm mass projects posteriorly from the left kidney. This mass is denser than the adjacent normal kidney. This was a hyperdense renal cyst.

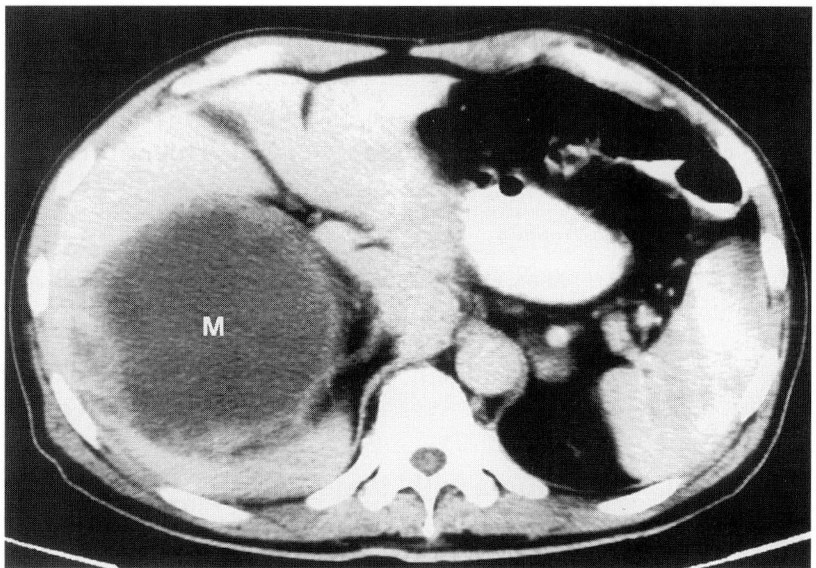

Figure 4–10. This right renal mass (M) has a density suggesting that it might be a simple cyst. However, the walls are slightly irregular. At surgery this was a cystic renal cell carcinoma.

or without wall nodules and mural or septal calcification that is not smooth. The walls may be thickened or irregular. This category includes lesions with a moderate probability of malignancy. Surgery is required for these lesions (Fig. 4–10). Category IV lesions have a cystic component but a nearly 100 percent probability of malignancy.

Incidental Renal Masses

As CT has become a common method of evaluating the abdomen, the incidentally discovered small renal mass has become commonplace. If the mass is less than 1 cm in diameter, measurement of density may be inaccurate due to volume averaging. With measurements of greater than 20 H, renal cell carcinoma becomes a possibility. Ultrasound is a logical next step in the evaluation of these lesions. If the lesion is cystic by ultrasound, the evaluation is complete. If the ultrasound shows something other than a cyst, CT scanning with and without contrast may solve the problem. Cuts 3 mm or 5 mm thick through the lesion are obtained, and multiple density measurements are made.

Contrast material must be administered in a controlled and precise manner. If scanning is performed in the corticomedullary phase, small lesions may be missed. The tubular phase is ideal for viewing the kidney. If a power injector is used and contrast material is injected at 2 mL/s, commencement of scanning at 90 seconds after the start of injection should allow good lesion detection. If the kidneys are scanned as part of a dynamic scan for liver evaluation, scanning will likely be performed during the corticomedullary phase and lesion detection will be suboptimal. In this situation, the kidneys can be quickly rescanned in a more optimal phase.

Magnetic resonance imaging performed both with and without gadolinium may be useful if the patient has renal insufficiency. This technique is as accurate as CT in detecting differential enhancement between mass and normal kidney.

Some lesions may be followed by repeat CT scans or repeat ultrasounds done every 6 months or even every year. This is safe because over 95 percent of renal cell carcinomas grow less than 1.3 cm per year and most renal cell carcinomas don't metastasize until they are at least 3 cm in size. Lesions above 1 cm in diameter (and therefore amenable to evaluation) should undergo ultrasound and/or CT evaluation. The ultrasound is done to prove or disprove the presence of a simple cyst; the CT to look for the fat of an angiomyolipoma. Echogenic lesions on ultrasound may not be angiomyolipomas. Small renal cell carcinomas may be echogenic.

Multiple Renal Masses

Multiple renal masses (Fig. 4–11) on any imaging study should suggest multiple cysts versus multiple neoplastic lesions. Metastases and lymphoma commonly present as multiple bilateral renal masses.

Subcapsular Hematoma with Tumor

Subcapsular hematomas around the kidney may be secondary to trauma, but consideration should always be given to other causes such as leaking aneurysms or renal, adrenal, or other retroperitoneal tumors. Vasculitis and renal infarcts can also lead to this finding. Acute hemorrhage usually has a high density and is homogeneous in appearance. It surrounds the kidney. The density is higher than the adjacent renal parenchyma. Over a matter of weeks, as the clot organizes and begins to dissolve, attenuation becomes more heterogeneous and approaches the attenuation of water. If the patient has a subcapsular or perirenal hematoma detected, but no tumor is seen, the patient should be reimaged after the hematoma has had time to completely resolve. The purpose of this is to make sure there is no small underlying tumor that has been obscured by the hemorrhagic area.

Spontaneous Perinephric Hemorrhage

Spontaneous perinephric hemorrhage may be the result of carcinoma or angiomyolipoma of the kidney. About one-third are caused by carcinoma and one-third by angiomyolipoma. Similar to subcapsular hematomas, spontaneous perinephric hemorrhage should be reimaged after time has been allowed for resolution of the hematoma to be certain that there is not an underlying tumor.

Angiomyolipomas

Angiomyolipomas are also known as renal hamartomas. These are benign tumors. Histologically, the tumor is composed of fat, smooth muscle, and thick-walled blood vessels (Fig. 4–12*A*). About 80 percent of these

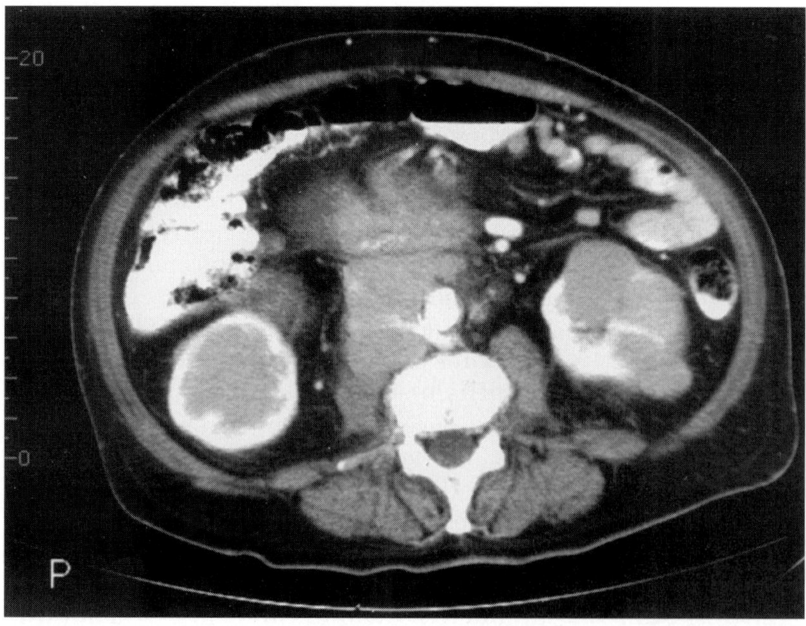

Figure 4–11. Multiple hypodense renal masses are present in both kidneys. These are secondary to renal lymphoma.

tumors occur sporadically, and another 20 percent are associated with tuberous sclerosis (Fig. 4–12*B*). They are more common in 40- to 60-year-old women. Patients can present with acute flank and abdominal pain due to hemorrhage, and occasionally can present with massive retroperitoneal hemorrhage causing shock. Hematuria is common. About 5 percent have calcification. The arteries in this tumor are disordered and frequently have aneurysms if angiography is performed. The diagnosis can be made by imaging if fat can be identified in the lesion.

The best imaging modalities to establish the diagnosis of angiomyolipoma are renal ultrasound, renal CT scanning, and renal MRI. At ultrasound, fat in the mass may

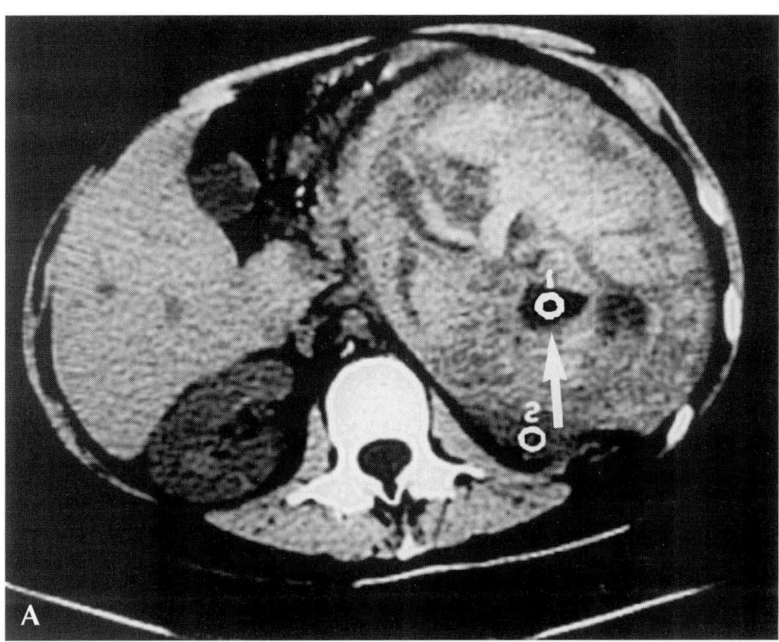

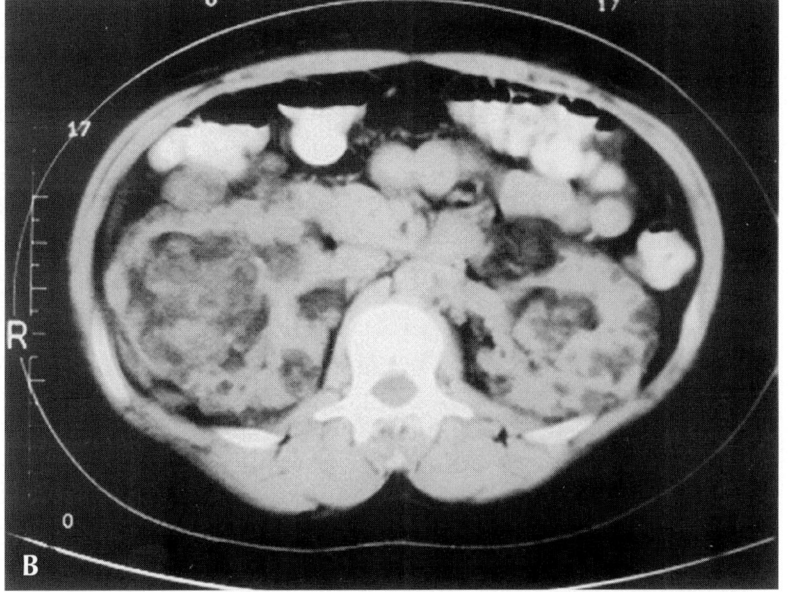

Figure 4–12. A. The fat (arrow) in this large heterogeneous left renal mass indicated an angiomyolipoma. This image is filmed in a narrow window to accentuate the detection of fat. **B.** Multiple areas of low density are present in both kidneys, indicating fat. This fat is due to the presence of multiple angiomyolipomas. This patient has tuberous sclerosis.

cause an area of increased echogenicity. Occasionally, adenocarcinomas may be highly echogenic so that the appearance on ultrasound is not specific.

Computer tomography is usually performed using thin cuts before the administration of intravenous contrast. Fat has a characteristic density, and when Hounsfield units are measured, fat will usually have a reading of approximately –80. Any reading below approximately 0 implies fat. About 95 percent of angiomyolipomas will have fat that can be identified by CT. If angiomyolipoma is suspected, a CT is the preferred way to evaluate the lesion.

The MRI evaluation of these tumors has been advocated to detect fat. Fat protons and water protons precess or spin at slightly different frequencies. If a tumor is scanned at TE = 4.4 mm/s and then scanned again at TE = 2.2 mm/s, the first scan will have fat and water in phase, and the signals from each pixel will be additive and therefore bright. At TE = 2.2 mm/s fat and water will be out of phase and the signal from fat will cancel the signal from water. Therefore, if fat is present, the signal will be decreased.

Transitional Cell Carcinoma of the Renal Pelvis

Less than 10 percent of malignant kidney tumors come from the uroepithelium. About 90 percent of these are transitional cell carcinomas (TCCs), and about 10 percent are squamous cell carcinomas. These tumors tend to be multicentric and bilateral. Metachronous and/or synchronous transitional cell carcinomas occur in up to 10 percent of patients. Patients with transitional cell carcinoma of the renal pelvis have a 7 percent chance of TCC on the other side and a 40 percent chance of developing transitional cell carcinoma of the bladder. Only 10 to 15 percent of TCCs develop in the upper tracts. A squamous cell carcinoma may develop from transitional cell epithelium that has undergone squamous metaplasia in response to chronic inflammation. Transitional cell carcinoma is more common in men, with a peak incidence in the seventh decade. Factors that increase the risk of development of this neoplasm include exposure to chemicals such as dyes, petroleum products, and products used in the rubber industry. Tobacco is a prominent inducer. Chronic inflammation and/or infection also increase the risk. The risk of this tumor is dramatically increased in patients who abuse analgesics, especially phenacetin. When squamous cell carcinoma occurs, it is in an older age group and is more likely to be associated with stones and chronic infection.

At imaging, these are mural lesions. A mural lesion will maintain a constant relationship with the renal pelvis or calyces despite changes in patient position. It should be partially surrounded by the contrast material. The lesion may be polypoid, sessile, or flat. It may be smooth or irregular. An intravenous urogram will detect about 60 to 70 percent of these tumors. If one filling defect is found, then a search for others should be made. If the tumor is large, then renal function may be impaired. If contrast material becomes trapped within a neoplastic mass, then a stippled appearance may be seen.

At CT, a mass that fills the collecting system and displaces the contrast material may be identified. The appearance on urography and CT (Fig. 4–13) is nonspecific and may be caused by other types of filling defects unless one can demonstrate with certainty that there is attachment to the wall. At ultrasound, the dense echoes from renal sinus fat may be displaced by a tumor. However, other causes of filling defects in the collecting system such as blood clots and fungus balls may have a similar appearance on an ultrasound exam. (Table 4–1).

At times, TCC of the renal pelvis may extend into the renal parenchyma and produce a focal parenchymal mass that may simulate an adenocarcinoma of the kidney. These TCCs usually infiltrate the kidney but maintain its reniform shape.

Filling Defects in the Ureter: Transitional Cell Carcinoma

Patients with transitional cell carcinoma of the ureter may have a synchronous transi-

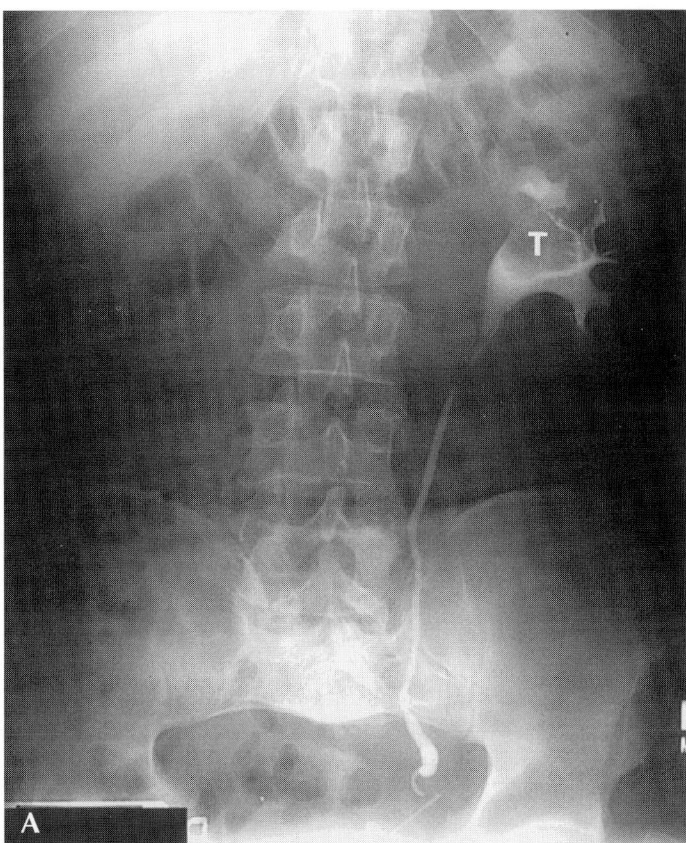

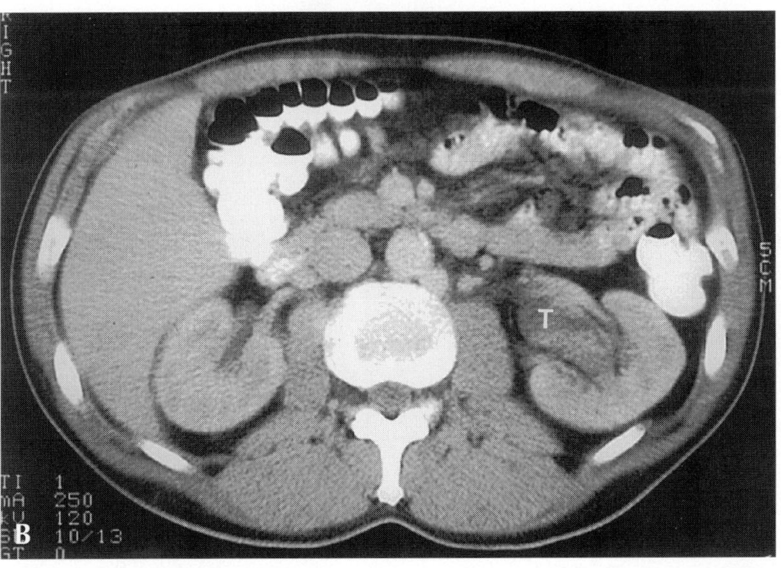

Figure 4–13. A. This retrograde study shows a filling defect from transitional cell carcinoma (T). **B.** A CT scan of the same patient shows a tumor (T) expanding the left renal pelvis.

tional cell carcinoma in 40 percent of cases. Transitional cell carcinoma of the bladder may develop in up to 55 percent of patients who have a ureteric lesion. The lower third of the ureter is involved in about two-thirds of patients, and the middle and upper thirds of the ureter are involved in about 15 percent of patients each. In excretory urogra-

TABLE 4–1. **Filling Defects in Renal Pelvis or Ureter**

Stones
Clots, mural hemorrhage
Debris from infection
Malakoplakia
Pus from pyelonephritis or instrumentation
Leukoplakia
Sloughed papillae
Pyelitis and ureteritis cystica
Fungus balls
Tumors
Transitional cell
Squamous cell
Adenocarcinoma
Fibroepithelial polyps
Metastases

phy, an intraluminal mass is seen, usually with obstruction of the ureter proximal to the mass. There may also be dilatation of the ureter distal to the mass. The cause of this is not known with certainty, but it may be to-and-fro peristalsis of the mass. This is known as the Bergman sign or goblet sign. The latter name comes from the fact that the tumor may cause an appearance resembling a chalice or goblet. The differential diagnosis of a filling defect in a ureter includes a stone. However, a stone usually causes spasm, not distention of the ureter distal to the filling defect. These tumors eventually lead to obstruction. Presenting symptoms include obstruction, but hematuria and metastatic disease are possibilities. An intravenous urogram will detect about 50 percent of ureteric tumors as filling defects (Fig. 4–14), 15 percent as hydronephrosis, and 5 percent as a mass. Transitional cell carcinomas can be staged using either the TNM system or the modified Jewett method (Table 4–2).

Retrograde pyelography is an important part of the workup and diagnosis of ureteral tumors (Fig. 4–15). Over 90 percent of TCCs

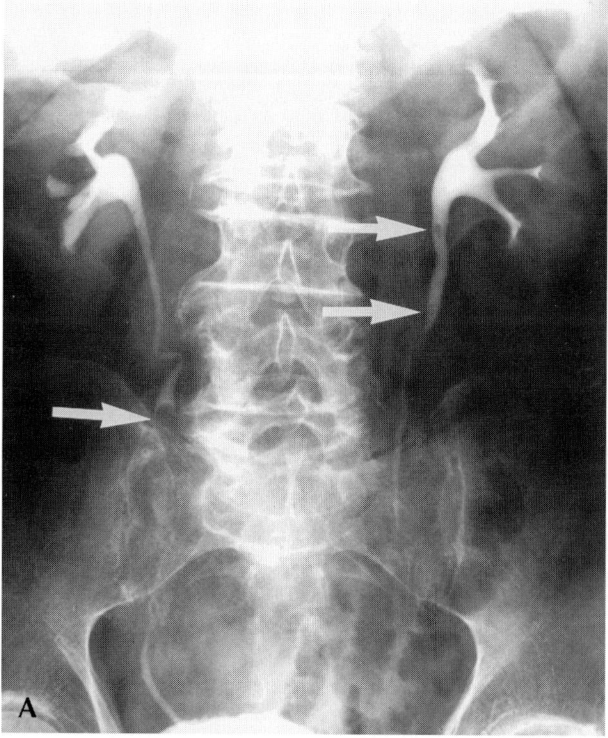

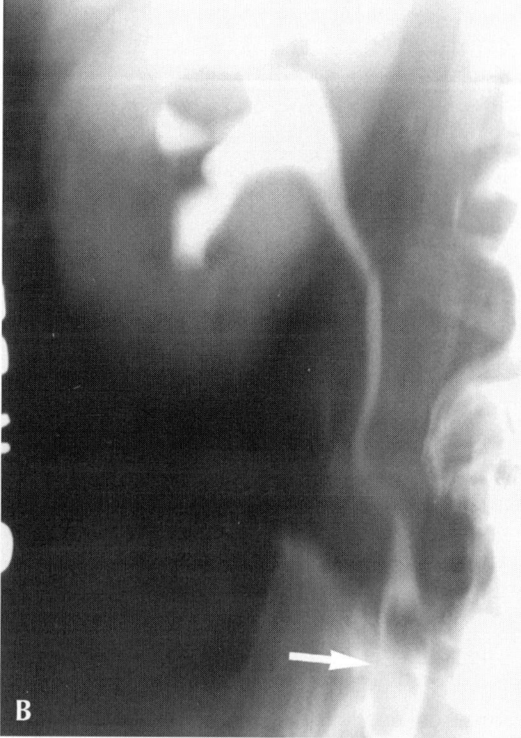

Figure 4–14. A. This urogram shows filling defects in the left proximal ureter (arrows) and a larger deficit in the right ureter (arrows). **B.** The defect in the right ureter (arrow) in a magnified image. These are transitional cell carcinomas.

TABLE 4–2. **Modified Jewett Staging**

Stage	Tumor	5-year Survival (%)
O	Mucosal only	100
A	Through lamina propria	80–95
B	Into muscular wall	40–80
C	Periureteral	15–30
D	Metastasized	0

will be detected by retrograde studies. This study is especially important in detecting coexistent urothelial tumors. Cytology can be obtained at the time that a retrograde urogram is done.

Wilm's Tumor

Wilm's tumor (Fig. 4–16) is the most common solid abdominal mass of childhood, with a peak incidence at about 36 months of age. Eighty percent occur before the age of 5. Fifteen percent of Wilm's tumors are associated with congenital abnormalities, including hemihypertrophy, sporadic nonfamilial aniridia, Beckwith-Wiedemann syndrome, pseudohermaphroditism (DRASH syndrome) (Fig. 4–16*C*), and neurofibromatosis. Deletion of the short arm of chromosome 11 is also associated with Wilm's tumor.

The tumor is often bulky, with a pseudocapsule separating it from adjoining normal kidney tissue (Fig. 4–16*C*). The tumor may appear cystic secondary to hemorrhage and necrosis. Wilm's tumor occasionally penetrates the renal capsule and is one of the tumors capable of invading the renal vein and IVC (Fig. 4–16*D*).

The staging of Wilm's tumor is as follows:

Stage I	Limited to kidney and excised with intact capsule.
Stage II	Tumor beyond kidney but resected; vessels outside kidney may be infiltrated. No tumor remaining after surgery. Tumor may extend locally into perirenal tissues.
Stage III	Lymph nodes positive, tumor spillage, or peritoneal implants beyond surgical margins.
Stage IV	Hematogenous metastasis.
Stage V	Bilateral renal involvement—stage each side.

Thirteen percent of Wilm's tumors are bilateral. Wilm's tumors may locally invade the tail of the pancreas, psoas muscle, diaphragm, splenic hilum, or porta hepatitis. The most common site of metastatic spread

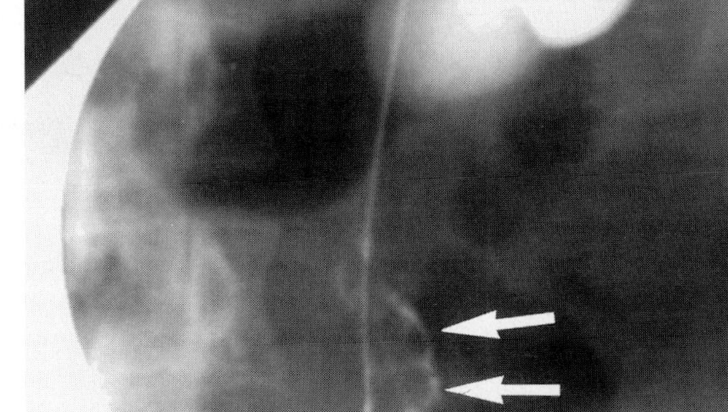

Figure 4–15. A retrograde ureterogram of the left side showing extensive transitional cell carcinoma (arrows).

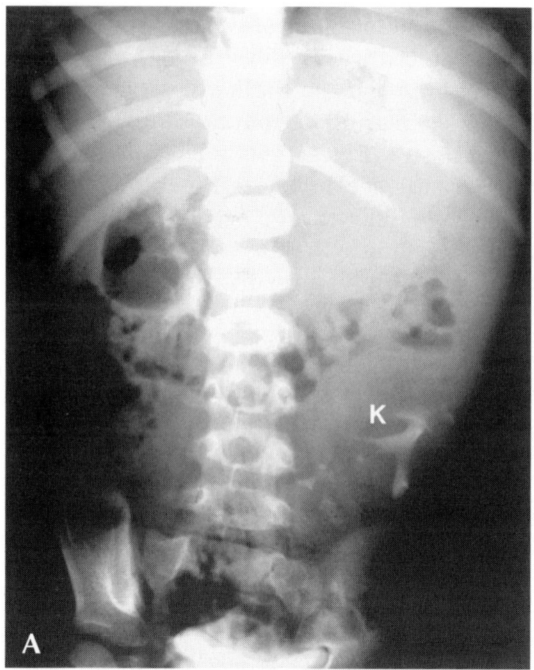

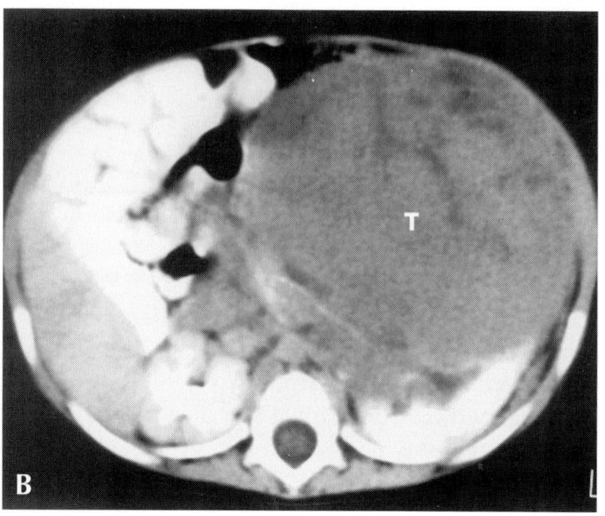

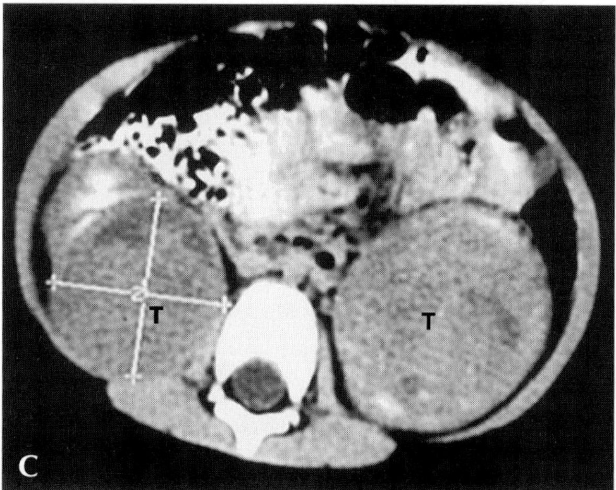

Figure 4–16. **A.** IVP. The Wilm's tumor has pushed the left kidney (K) down. **B.** CT in the same patient shows the huge mass of a Wilm's tumor (T). **C.** DRASH syndrome with bilateral Wilm's tumors. **D.** Wilm's tumor with a tumor clot (T) in the inferior vena cava.

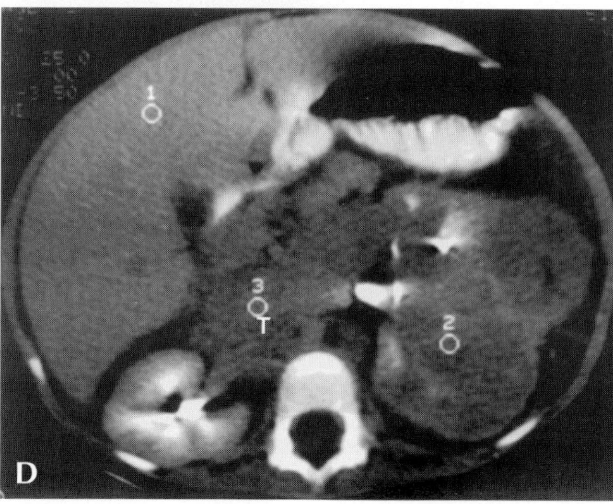

is to the lungs, with the liver being second. As mentioned, Wilm's tumor may invade the IVC, extend to the heart, or invade caudally through gonadal veins.

Plain film findings of Wilm's tumor include a bulging flank (75 percent), loss of renal or psoas outline, renal enlargement, and bowel gas displacement. Ten percent will have abdominal calcification. On IVU, the kidney is enlarged. Normal excretion of contrast is present in 75 percent. Twenty percent will have only a nephrogram or delayed filling of the collecting system, and 5 percent will show no contrast material excretion. If the kidney functions, calyces are often distorted.

Ultrasound shows a well-defined mass, which has a variable echo pattern. There may be areas of hyper- or hypoechogenicity, reflecting fat or necrosis. Computed tomography shows a well-defined mass with lower density than adjacent normal tissue (Fig. 4–16*B–D*). Mild enhancement of the tumor is usually seen. Fat and/or calcification also may be seen. The tumor is usually heterogeneous in appearance. On MRI, the signal intensity is variable because of necrosis and hemorrhage. In general, nonnecrotic portions of the tumor show a low signal on T1 and a high signal on T2 sequences.

In a child with a suspected abdominal mass, ultrasound is the screening test of choice. If ultrasound shows a mass, then CT should be the next test for characterization and evaluation of extent. We prefer MRI for evaluation of caval extension and extension to the heart.

Once a patient with Wilm's tumor has been treated, follow-up imaging should be limited to the chest and abdomen by CT. These follow-up studies may cease after 2 years.

Patients who are at high risk for developing Wilm's tumor, such as those with sporadic aniridia (up to 33 percent incidence), hemihypertrophy, or Beckwith syndrome should be followed with periodic ultrasound exams.

Nephroblastomatosis refers to the presence of embryonal renal tissue. These clusters have also been called nephrogenic rests. Patients with nephroblastomatosis have an increased incidence of development of Wilm's tumor. However, most of these nephrogenic rests do not develop into Wilm's tumors. The rests appear on IVP as nonspecific masses with calyceal displacement. On ultrasound these masses are hypo- or isoechoic. On CT, the rests enhance poorly after contrast and are of lower density than adjacent kidney. Children with rests should be followed with ultrasound every 3 months until the age of 4.

Neuroblastoma

Neuroblastoma is discussed here because of its similarity to Wilm's tumor. Neuroblastoma originates from neural tissue, frequently the adrenal gland. It occurs at a slightly younger age than Wilm's tumor (50 percent under 2, 75 percent under 4 years). These patients commonly present with a palpable abdominal mass (about 50 percent), and they also present with pain and fever (30 percent), bone pain, limp or inability to walk (20 percent), myoclonus, cerebellar ataxia, or nystagmus. Neuroblastoma is not linked to other syndromes or genetic disease.

Plain films of neuroblastoma may show a mass effect, and about 50 percent of neuroblastomas will have stippled or mottled calcifications. Computed tomography is the method of choice for delineating the extent of the tumor and whether or not surrounding structures have been invaded. At ultrasound, an extrarenal mass will be seen displacing the kidney in a caudad direction. The tumor is usually solid and the echo appearance ranges from hyperechoic to hypoechoic. It is a poorly defined tumor with a heterogeneous appearance. Shadowing secondary to the calcification may be seen.

At CT, the lesion is usually of soft tissue density with well-defined margins. About 90 percent have calcification on CT. The tumor may be homogeneous or heterogeneous. Patchy enhancement occurs after contrast. On MRI, most neuroblastomas have a high signal on T2-weighted images. Intravenous urography should not be used in the evaluation of neuroblastoma. At ultrasound neuroblastoma is quite variable in appearance. The tumor is frequently of intermediate echogenicity, but necrotic areas may be low

TABLE 4–3. **International Staging System for Neuroblastoma**

Stage	Description
1	• Localized tumor confined to the area of origin • Complete gross excision with or without microscopic residual disease • Identifiable ipsilateral and contralateral lymph nodes negative microscopically
2A	• Unilateral tumor with incomplete gross excision • Identifiable ipsilateral and contralateral lymph nodes negative microscopically
2B	• Unilateral tumor with complete or incomplete gross excision • Unilateral tumor with positive ipsilateral regional lymph nodes • Identifiable contralateral lymph nodes negative microscopically
3	• Tumor infiltrating across the midline with or without regional lymph node involvement • Or, unilateral tumor with contralateral regional lymph node involvement • Or, midline tumor with bilateral regional lymph node involvement
4	• Dissemination of tumor to distant lymph nodes, bone, bone marrow, liver, or other organs (except as defined in stage 4S)
4S	• Localized primary tumor as defined for stage 1 or 2 with dissemination limited to liver, skin, or bone marrow

in echogenicity. Shadowing secondary to calcifications is often visible.

Neuroblastoma may be found in any location where there are tissues of the sympathetic nervous system. Tumor in the adrenal medulla is common (40 percent of cases), and this leads to the confusion with Wilm's tumor.

There are several staging schemes for neuroblastoma. The International Staging System is listed in Table 4–3.

Because of bone involvement in Stages 4 and 4S, the workup of bone metastases requires bone scanning. Bone scanning is significantly more sensitive for skeletal metastases than plain films. The primary tumor may also take up the bone scanning agent in up to 75 percent of cases.

Chapter

5

Inflammatory Conditions of the Upper Tract

ACUTE PYELONEPHRITIS

Acute pyelonephritis is an acute bacterial infection of the kidney. It is common in women between 15 and 30 years old. These patients present with fever, flank pain, and white blood cells and bacteria in the urine. Acute pyelonephritis usually develops from an ascending bacterial infection that initially seeded the bladder. Bacteria reach the region of the medullary rays, and an inflammatory response develops. The inflammatory response causes debris to fill the tubules. The most common organism is *Escherichia coli,* although *Proteus mirabilis* is also a common agent. Imaging is indicated only when the clinical diagnosis is in doubt or there has been a poor response to antibiotics. A history of stones or diabetes mellitus may also be indications for imaging.

On imaging studies, the kidney becomes diffusely enlarged (Fig. 5–1*A*). The kidney will not concentrate contrast material as well as the nonaffected kidney, and there is delayed opacification of the calyces and pelvis. Overall, the kidney is less dense after the administration of intravenous contrast than the normal kidney. Occasional swelling of one of the poles may be seen, with dilatation of either the renal pelvis or calyces. On CT, the abnormality may be limited to wedge-shaped zones in the kidney, which will have less density than the surrounding kidney (Fig. 5–1*B*). Computed tomography scanning should not be performed in the corticomedullary phase (30 to 60 seconds after the start of contrast imaging) but instead should be done during the tubular phase (75 to 120 seconds after the start of contrast imaging) because this phase is more sensitive for the changes of infection. Occasionally, patchy or poorly defined defects may be seen. At ultrasound there may be diffuse renal enlargement. The area of infection may have either increased or, as is more common, decreased echogenicity, probably secondary to the edema associated with infection.

Emphysematous pyelonephritis is a gas-forming infection of the kidney that occurs predominantly in diabetics. These patients are acutely ill, with an elevated white blood cell count, pyuria, fever, and flank pain. Mortality is high. This disease is usually considered an emergency requiring urgent nephrectomy, although some cases may be treated with antibiotics. Patients with gas in the collecting system have a better prognosis than those with gas in the parenchyma. Gas also may be seen within the interstitium of

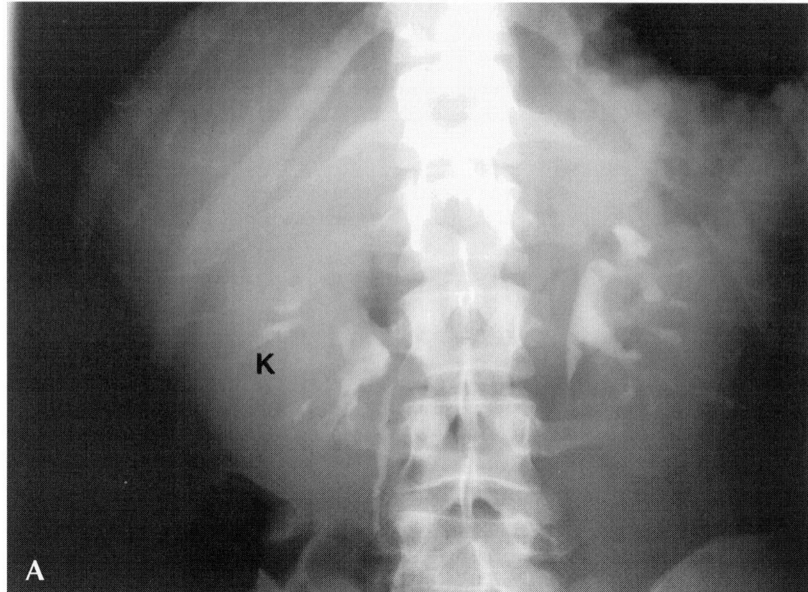

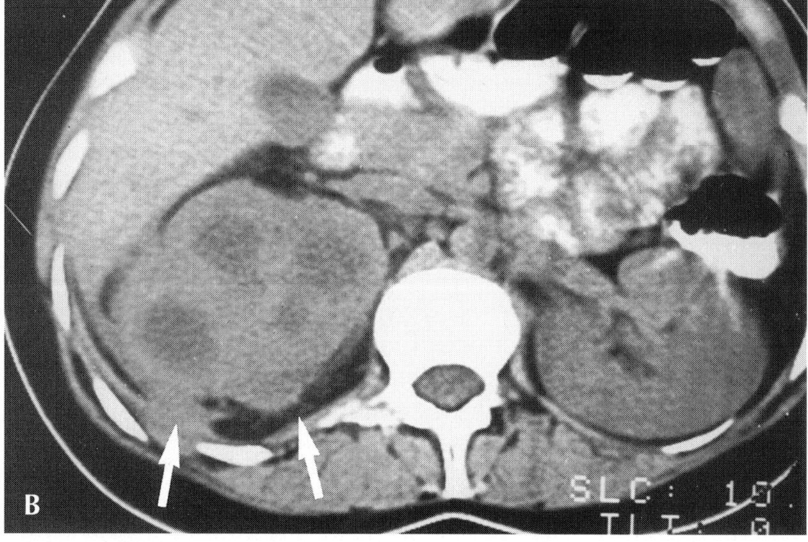

Figure 5–1. A. Acute pyelonephritis of right kidney (K). The kidney is diffusely enlarged. The calyces are spread and are not as well opacified as those of the left kidney. **B.** CT scan without contrast material. The right kidney is enlarged. Multiple low-density areas are seen within the kidney. Inflammatory stranding is present around the kidney (arrows).

the kidney or even the perinephric space, and may extend throughout the retroperitoneum (Fig. 5–2). On intravenous urography, the kidney may be nonfunctional but a plain film may reveal a gas shadow in the shape of the kidney. Ultrasound sometimes shows echogenic foci due to gas bubbles. Ultrasound is not as sensitive as CT in detecting the gas in the kidney.

Acute infection, which involves only a limited portion of the kidney, may produce a mass effect secondary to edema (Fig. 5–3). Terms such as *acute bacterial nephritis, lobar nephronia, focal bacterial nephritis, carbuncle, renal cellulitis,* and *renal phlegmon* have been used. The Society of Uroradiology currently recommends that *acute pyelonephritis with focal swelling* is the appropriate descriptor.

Cortical scintigraphy with technetium-99m DMSA has been used in children with acute pyelonephritis to determine renal parenchymal involvment. Positive scans show focal regions of decreased uptake with a sensitivity of about 90 percent.

Renal ultrasound for acute pyelonephritis is mainly used to exclude obstruction, stones, and abscesses. Ultrasound has a

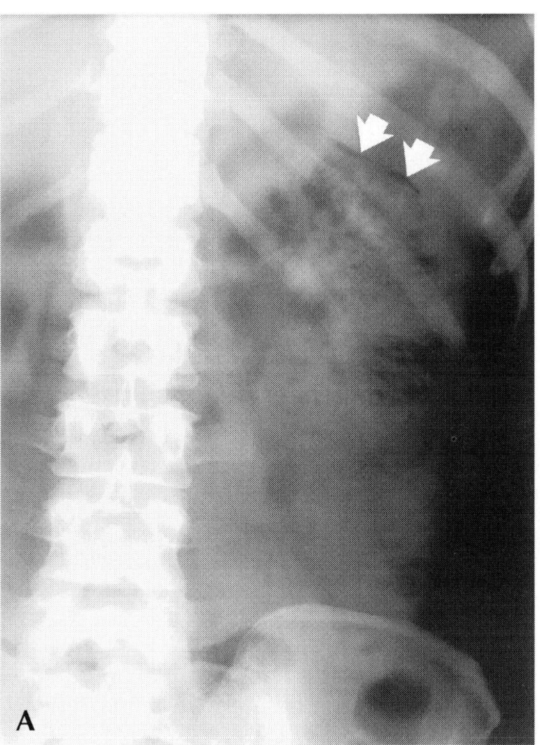

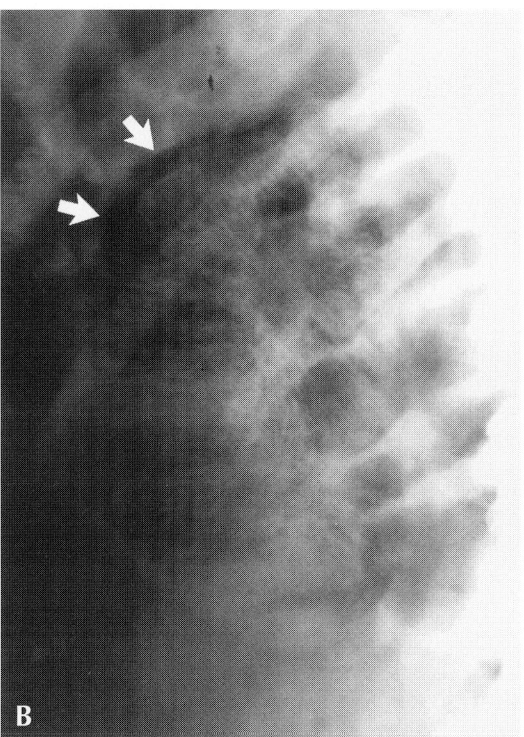

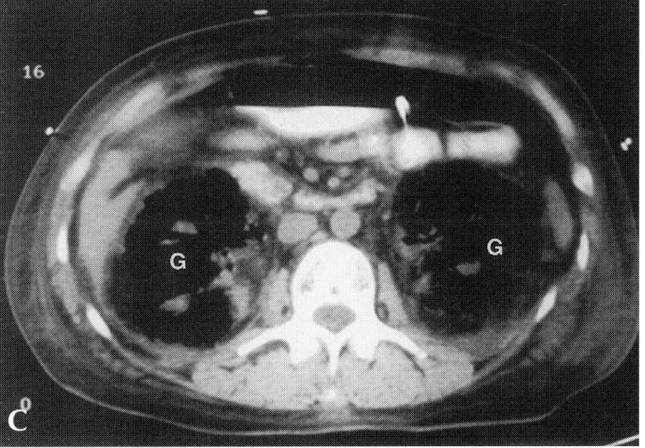

Figure 5–2. A. Emphysematous pyelonephritis of the left kidney. Gas is present within the renal parenchyma. A small rim of gas (arrows) outlines the upper pole. **B.** A different patient with emphysematous pyelonephritis. There is gas within the parenchyma and a rim of gas outlining the kidney (arrows). **C.** A CT scan of bilateral emphysematous pyelonephritis with gas (G) within the kidneys. **D.** Gas within the calyces.

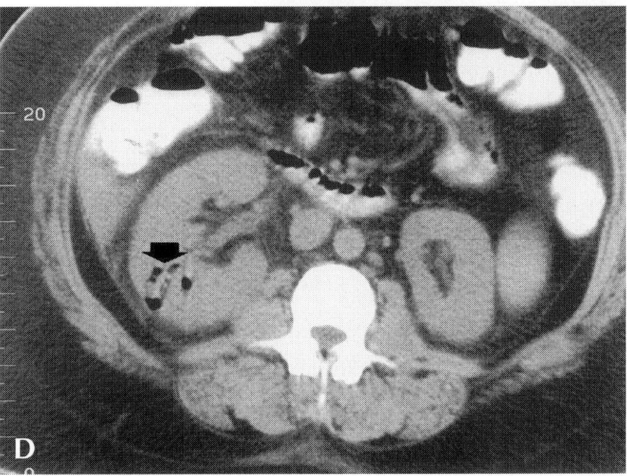

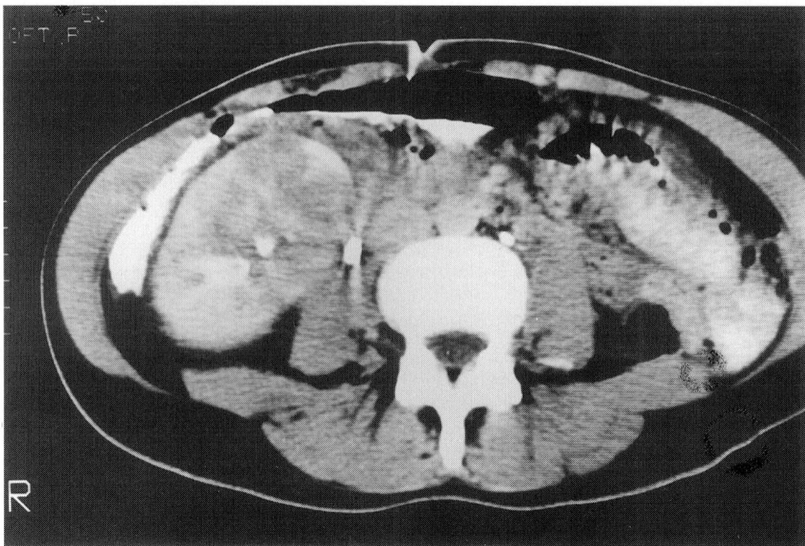

Figure 5–3. Acute pyelonephritis with focal swelling. The anterior right kidney is focally enlarged with patchy areas of nonenhancement.

sensitivity of less than 50 percent in diagnosing acute pyelonephritis and is not as good as CT at detecting abscesses. Power Doppler of the kidneys has recently been shown to increase the sensitivity of ultrasound, however. Intravenous urography has not been as widely used in the routine imaging of suspected pyelonephritis since the introduction of ultrasound as a more minimally invasive procedure.

CORTICAL ABSCESS

A renal abscess presents with symptoms of pyelonephritis. An abscess occurs when foci of pyelonephritis coalesce into an area of infection with secondary necrosis. A renal abscess is more likely to form when the ureter or renal pelvis is obstructed. Unlike acute pyelonephritis, which is more common in females, males are more likely to develop a renal abscess. Patients with a history of immunodeficiency are also more likely to develop an abscess.

Imaging of a cortical abscess by excretory urography may reveal an indistinct renal outline. The margin of the psoas muscle may also be blurred. The collecting system may be attenuated by a unifocal mass. There may even be a lucent area in the center of the mass. On renal CT there will be less enhancement of the abscess compared to the remaining normal kidney. The CT density of the central portion of the abscess may equal that of water. Rupture into the perinephric space is easily detected with CT. On nonenhanced scans, it may be difficult to see an abscess if the density is identical to that of the adjacent renal parenchyma. Therefore, intravenous contrast material should be administered. At ultrasound, a focal mass will be identified with mixed echogenicity. The central portion will usually be hypoechoic secondary to the necrosis and water-like consistency of the abscess. The walls may be irregular, and there may be some through transmission of sound.

PERINEPHRIC ABSCESS

A perinephric abscess occurs when a renal abscess is incompletely walled off and the abscess penetrates the renal capsule to infiltrate the perinephric space within Gerota's fascia. A perinephric abscess may also occur when infected urine extravasates as a result of pyelosinus backflow. An infection may be spread hematogenously from another infected organ. Finally, a perinephric abscess may form by direct extension into the perinephric space from adjacent organs, such as bowel or appendix. The presenting symptoms are very similar to those of pyelonephritis or renal abscess. It is not uncommon for the urinalysis to be normal.

Intravenous urography of an perinephric abscess may show a soft-tissue-density mass extending laterally from the kidney. The margins of the kidney may be blurred.

On CT, perinephric abscess appears as a mixed-density, soft tissue mass surrounding the kidney in the perinephric space. There may be extension to involve the psoas muscle. Gas may be present in the abscess.

Ultrasound will show a mixed echogenicity mass surrounding or adjacent to the kidney. If gas is present, it will sometimes be identified as acoustic shadowing with a ring-down artifact.

PYONEPHROSIS

Pyonephrosis is infected hydronephrosis. This may quickly lead to cortical and perinephric abscesses. Xanthogranulomatous pyelonephritis and/or fistulae to bowel or pleura may develop. At ultrasound, hydronephrosis is seen but fine low-level echoes, representing debris, may be seen within the fluid. However, ultrasound is only about 50 percent sensitive for these echoes. At CT, the debris in the fluid may not be visible and the appearance may be that of hydronephrosis.

XANTHOGRANULOMATOUS PYELONEPHRITIS

Xanthogranulomatous pyelonephritis (XGP) is a disease that predominantly affects middle-aged or older females, although it may occur in children and young adults. These patients usually have chronic undiagnosed urinary tract infection with either *E. coli* or *P. mirabilis.* Classically, these patients have a staghorn calculus, absent or decreased excretion of contrast material at intravenous urography, and a renal mass. They may have abdominal and flank pain and signs of infection, including weight loss and anemia. About 75 percent of the cases will have an obstructing stone in the renal pelvis, and frequently this is a staghorn type of calculus. Histologically, there are lipid-laden macrophages as well as all types of inflammatory cells, including plasma cells and white blood cells.

Xanthogranulomatous pyelonephritis has been broken down into a focal form and a diffuse form. The focal form is frequently referred to as tumefactive xanthogranulomatous pyelonephritis. This tumefactive form leads to a masslike configuration involving only a portion of the kidney and resembles a neoplasm. The diffuse form involves the whole kidney.

Plain films often show a staghorn calculus and may show a poorly defined mass. After administration of contrast there is usually poor excretion of the contrast material (Fig. 5–4*A*). Many cases will have hydronephrosis. At renal CT, the kidney is usually diffusely enlarged and calculi are usually seen (Fig. 5–4*B-D*). There may be low-density areas consistent with necrosis or obstruction of calyces. The tissue at the periphery of the obstructed calyces may enhance very intensely, possibly due to the inflammatory reaction. This disease sometimes extends into the perinephric space and on into adjacent organs, leading to a widespread inflammatory mass.

Ultrasound shows an irregularly enlarged kidney with multiple dilated calyces. These may have internal echoes consistent with the debris within them. The calculus can usually be identified as a highly reflective structure with a shadow behind it. Retrograde pyelography shows a contracted distorted pelvis with filling defects secondary to xanthogranulomas.

FUNGUS

Patients who have a history of diabetes, immunocompromise, or intraveneous drug use are at increased risk for fungal infec-

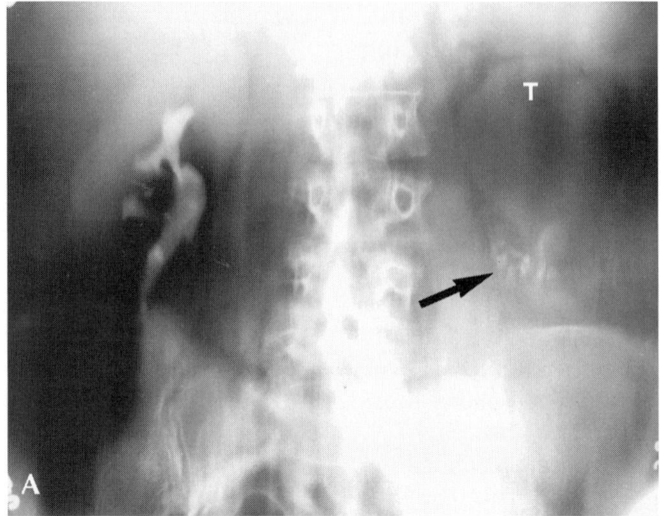

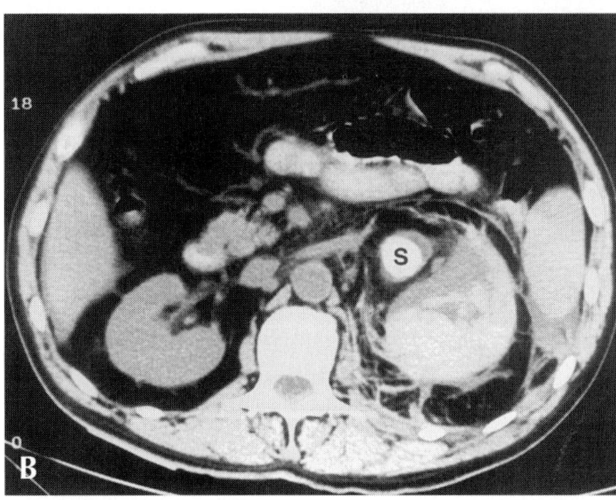

Figure 5–4. Xanthogranulomatous pyelonephritis. **A.** An intravenous urogram showing poor enhancement and excretion of contrast material by the left kidney, a tumefactive swelling of the upper pole (T), and stones in the region of the left renal pelvis (arrow). **B.** CT in a different patient shows a staghorn calculus on the left (S), swelling of the left kidney, and patchy enhancement of the left kidney. **C.** CT of right xanthogranulomatous pyelonephritis with swelling, a staghorn calculus (S) and a low-density area within the kidney. **D.** Right xanthogranulomatous pyelonephritis with focal low-density areas, swelling, and a calculus. The left kidney is also abnormal, with severe hydronephrosis and a very thin cortex.

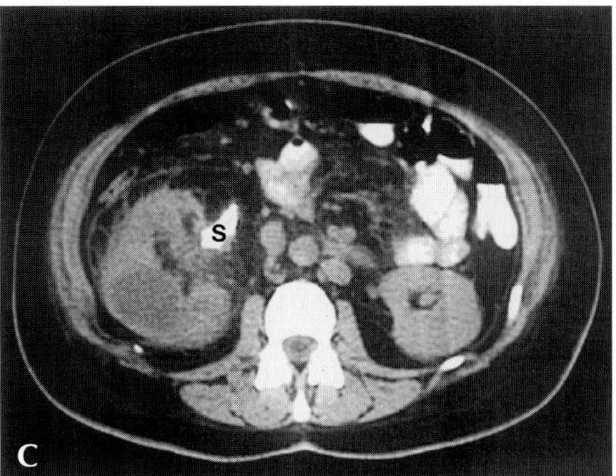

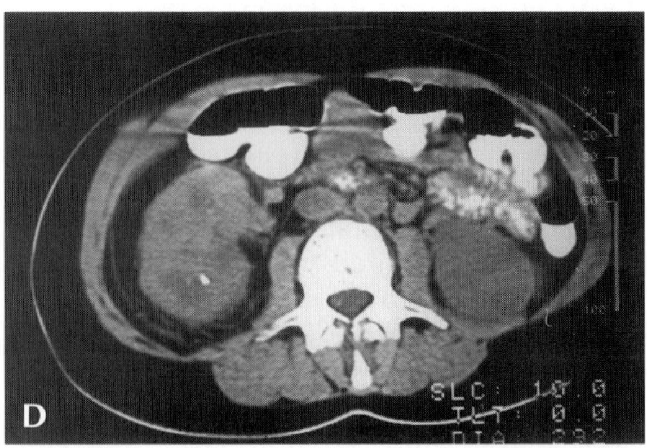

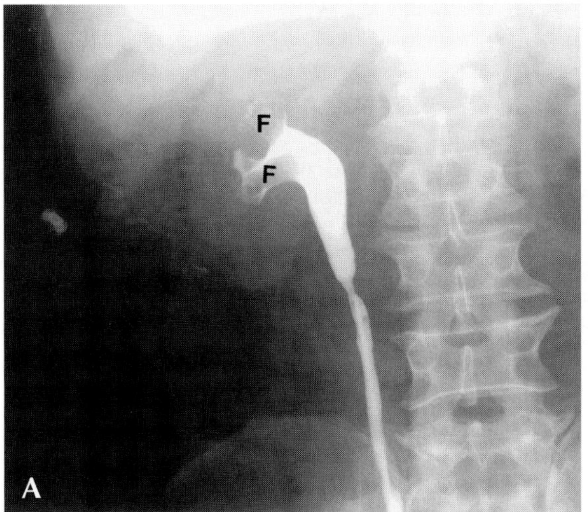

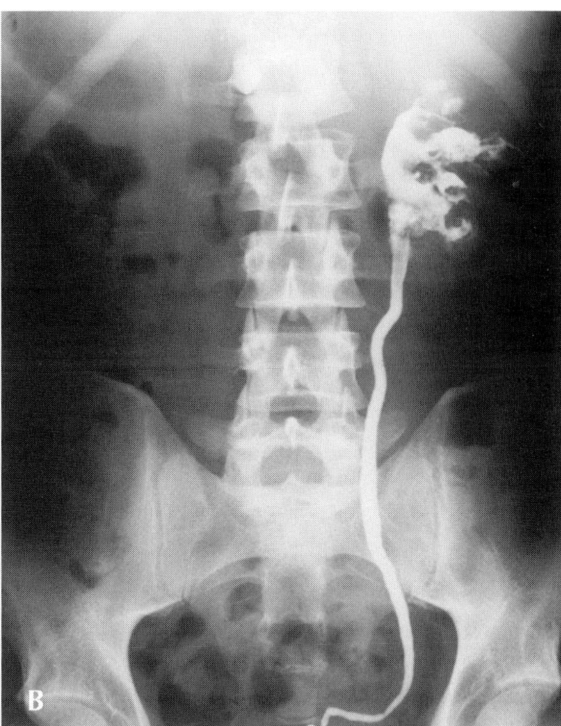

Figure 5–5. A. An intravenous urogram with fungus balls (F). **B.** A retrograde study in aspergillosis. The pelvis and calyces are irregular and distorted.

tion. Premature infants undergoing intensive care are also at risk. Candida is the most common pathogen, but aspergillus, coccidioides, cryptococcus, actinomycosis, nocardia, and mucormycosis are also seen. Filling defects occur secondary to fungus balls (mycetomas) and their associated debris. Obstruction or destruction of the kidney may result (Fig. 5–5).

TUBERCULOSIS

Tuberculosis (TB) of the urinary tract occurs as a result of hematogenous spread of *Mycobacterium tuberculosis* from a distant site, usually the lungs. However, only about 50 percent of patients have chest x-ray evidence of either active or inactive tuberculosis at the time that urologic TB is diagnosed. Only 10 percent of patients will have active disease at the time urologic tuberculosis is diagnosed. The hematogenous dissemination results in lesions in both kidneys. Most of these lesions heal, and renal tuberculosis is commonly a unilateral process. Renal or urologic tuberuculosis is an indolent disease. Lower urinary tract symptoms such as frequency and dysuria are the most common complaint on presentation. Fever, malaise, and other generalized symptoms are not as common. After seeding of the kidney, the tuberculosis bacterium moves along the nephron and ultimately ruptures into the collecting system (i.e., the calyx).

At urography, the earliest finding is irregularity of either the papillae or calyces. Ultimately, papillary necrosis may occur, leading to large cavities in the kidney. These lesions in the kidney tend to calcify (Fig. 5–6). Eventually, the kidney functions poorly and may even become nonfunctional. Frank autonephrectomy may occur. Infundibular stenoses or strictures are common. If stenosis of the infundibulum is severe enough, the calyx may be cut off from the remainder of the collecting system and

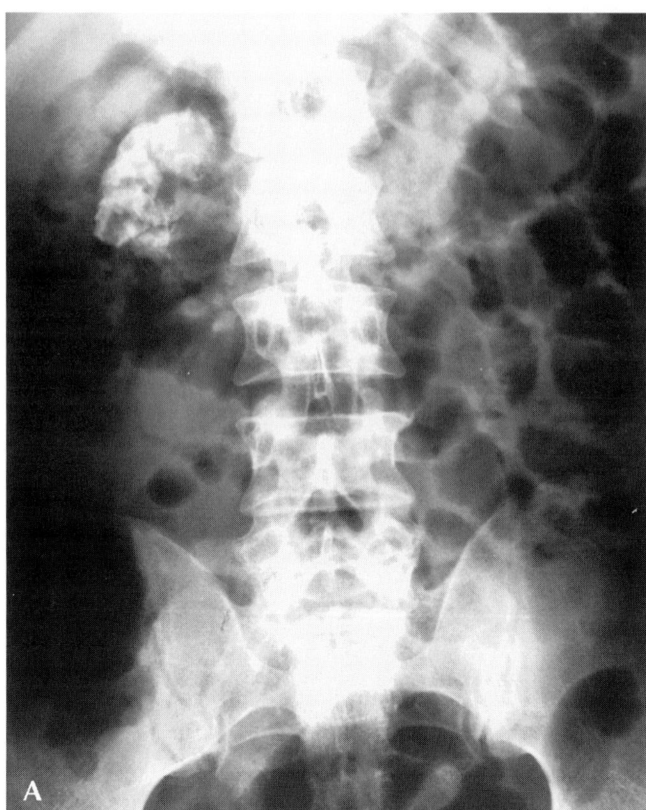

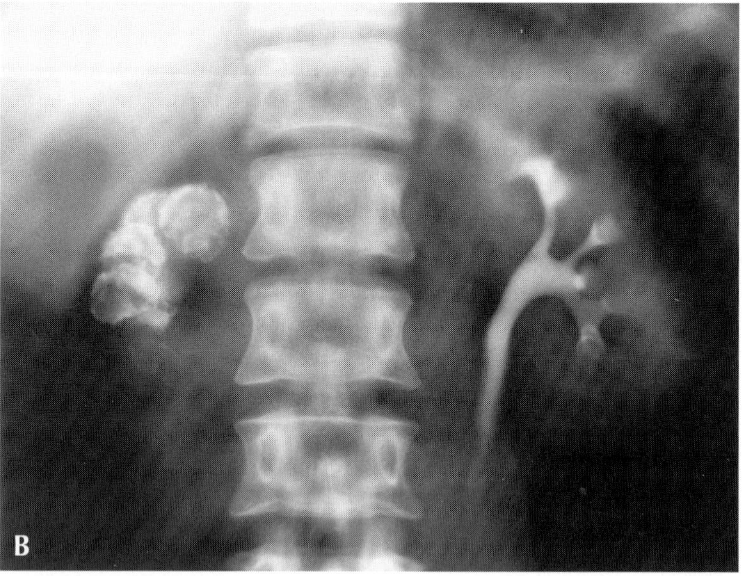

Figure 5–6. A. Plain film showing a calcified cavity within the right kidney from tuberculosis. **B.** A tomogram from an intravenous urogram in the same patient shows that the right kidney is nonfunctioning. The majority of the kidney is calcified.

may not opacify. As the granulomas in the kidney grow and merge, masslike lesions form. The kidney becomes distorted. As these masses rupture into the collecting system, a cavity may be left.

The ureter ultimately may have multiple strictures with areas of dilatation (Fig. 5–7). Tuberculous strictures of the ureter tend to occur at the infundibula, ureteropelvic junction and in the distal ureters. The bladder may be thick-walled and irregular. Calcification of either the epididymis or the seminal

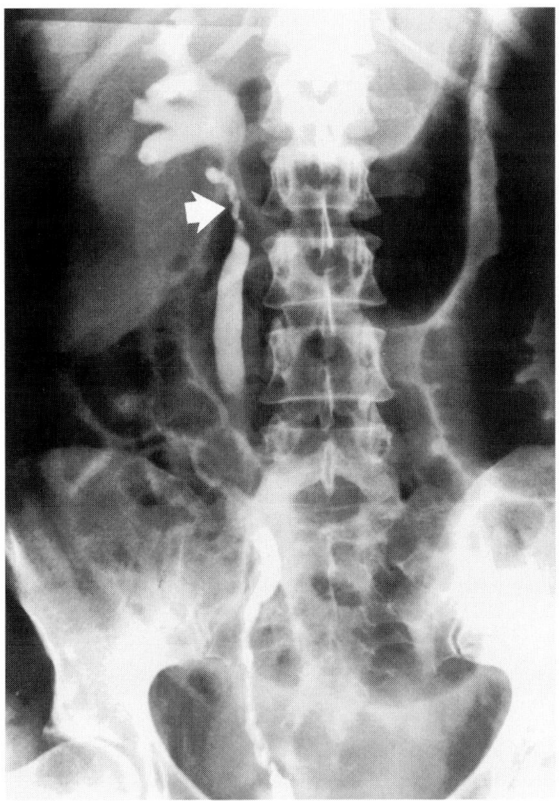

Figure 5–7. Ureteric tuberculosis. This retrograde study shows extensive stricture formation in the right proximal ureter (arrow).

vesicle may sometimes be seen. At both ultrasound and CT, calcifications are seen with irregularity of the margin of the kidney. The kidney may be normal in size, small, or even large if hydronephrosis is present. After contrast material is administered, enhancement may be diminished if there has been significant renal damage. The calyces, infundibula, and renal pelvis may be distorted, with areas of narrowing. Areas of low density may be present due to necrosis or debris-laden calyces. On CT, calcification of the ureters may be seen.

VESICOURETERAL REFLUX AND REFLUX NEPHROPATHY

The term *chronic pyelonephritis* has been a confusing term, and the term currently preferred is *chronic atrophic pyelonephritis* or *reflux nephropathy*. Reflux nephropathy occurs as a result of the reflux of infected urine from the bladder into the renal tubules. Intrarenal reflux into the papilla and into the tubules may occur as a result of high pressures in the collecting system.

The papilla normally has a slitlike orifice to prevent intrarenal reflux. However, distortion of this configuration due to hydronephrosis may cause reflux through these openings into the papillary ducts, especially at the upper and lower poles. Intrarenal reflux then causes parenchymal scarring, which extends throughout the thickness of the renal cortex. This is true even though the disease process is initially centered in the medulla.

In response to the scarring and retraction of the papillary process, the calyx becomes widened. Therefore, the radiologic findings of a chronic atrophic pyelonephritis or reflux nephropathy typically show scars at either the upper pole or the lower pole of the kidney with a deformed calyx (Fig. 5–8). Adjacent to the deformed calyx, the cortex may show evidence of compensatory hypertrophy. On ultrasound there will be a focal loss of renal parenchyma consistent with a scar. Increased focal echogenicity in the area of the scar may also be apparent. It is currently thought that the refluxed urine must be infected to cause reflux nephropathy. There is debate as to whether or not sterile urine that refluxes can cause reflux nephropathy. The earliest lesion of reflux nephropathy is an acute segmental or lobar nephritis. Usually this is not imaged, but if it is, there may be a focal enlargement of the kidney in the involved area. A nephrogram may show decreased density, and ultrasound will show either increased or decreased echogenicity. Technetium-99m DMSA has been used to detect areas of scarring because scar tissue will not bind this substance but normal nephrons will.

Because vesicoureteral reflux is such a potential source of renal parenchymal damage, urinary tract infections are usually evaluated with voiding cystourethrography. The ureters are watched fluoroscopically while the child voids. Film detection of reflux is more sensitive than detection on a fluoroscopic monitor, so films are usually

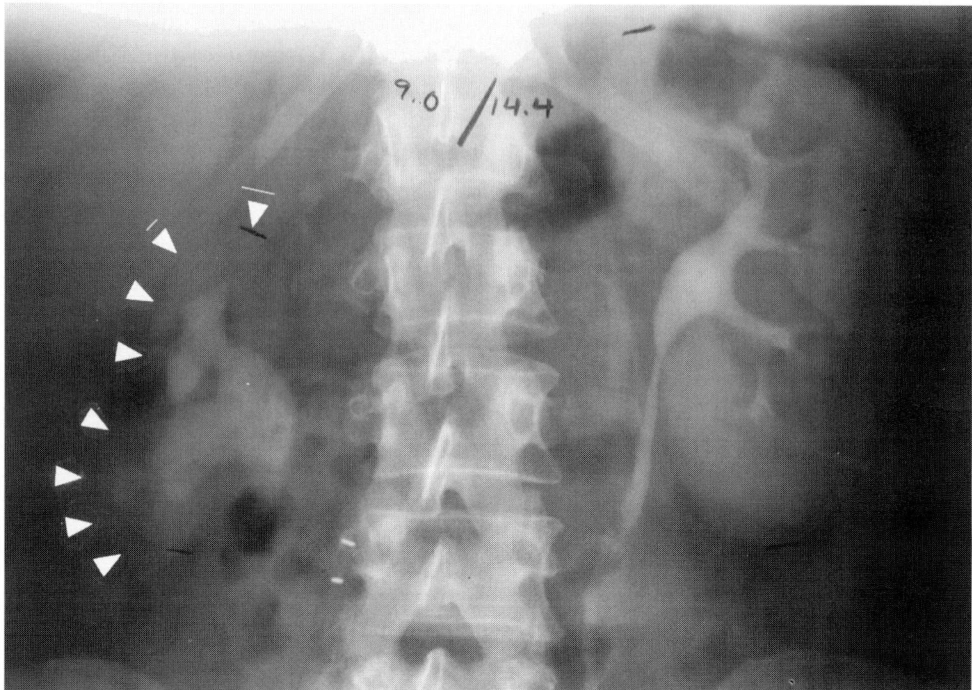

Figure 5–8. Reflux nephropathy. The right kidney is outlined by arrowheads. The calyces are widened. The cortex is thin and irregular, especially near the upper-pole calyces, indicating scarring. There is compensatory hypertrophy of the left kidney.

also obtained while the child voids. Reflux is graded by the following: Grade 1, ureter only; Grade 2, ureter, pelvis, and calyces without dilatation and with normal fornices; Grade 3, ureter, pelvis, and calyces with mild dilatation but normal fornices; Grade 4, ureter, pelvis, and calyces with moderate dilatation/tortuosity, deformed or unsharp fornices, and normal papillae; Grade 5, gross distention with effaced papillae.

At ultrasound, reflux into calyces (Grade 3) may occasionally be seen. This is manifested by dilatation of the calyces. However, many patients who reflux will not have an episode of reflux during the ultrasound exam. If the kidney is damaged and scarred, then it will be small with increased echogenicity. Medullary hyperechogenicity is an indicator of reflux that may be seen before scarring. Finally, the contour of the kidney may be irregular secondary to cortical scars.

PAPILLARY NECROSIS

Papillary necrosis occurs secondary to ischemia of the renal papillae. There is resultant partial or complete necrosis of these papillae. The papilla is sloughed into the collecting system and may produce obstruction. The most common cause is analgesic nephropathy. In the past, this was usually due to phenacetin, but currently it may be due to combinations of aspirin, acetaminophen, and other nonsteroidal anti-inflammatory agents. A popular mnemonic for remembering the most common causes of papillary necrosis is POSTCARD (P = pyelonephritis, O = obstruction, S = sickle cell disease, T = tuberculosis, C = cirrhosis, A = analgesics, R = renal vein thrombosis, D = diabetes). Other causes include prolonged hypotension, urinary tract obstruction, dehydration, hematuria, and cirrhosis. Papillary necrosis is most common in middle-aged to elderly women. The symptoms resemble those of a urinary tract infection. There may be cavitation of the central part of the renal papillae, which is sometimes referred to as medullary or partial papillary slough. If the entire renal papillae sloughs, then this is referred to as total papillary sloughing. The sloughed portion of the renal papillae produces urinary tract obstruction. When necrotic tissue does pass down the collecting system, it is usually radiolucent and can be appreciated only by the obstructed column of contrast material. It can not be distinguished from blood clots.

Radiographically, the kidneys are usually normal in size. In more severe cases the kidneys will become small. The kidney contour is usually smooth. After intravenous contrast has been administered, a line of contrast material will be seen extending from the calyx into the parenchyma of the kidney. This corresponds to the cavity in the renal papillae (Fig. 5–9). Nephrocalcinosis may be seen, especially in cases caused by analgesic abuse. There are foci of calcification corresponding to the papillae tips. Over time, progressive renal failure may occur, with inability of the kidney to adequately concentrate the contrast material. The findings on CT scanning are similar to those on plain films, with calcifications near the papillary tip prior to contrast material administration and contrast material extending into a cavity in the papillary tip after contrast material administration. Overall, ultrasound is not sensitive for this condition. Stones or calcifications may be appreciated in the region of the papillary tip. Calyces may be dilated if there is obstruction. The papillary calcification is more common in necrosis secondary to analgesic abuse.

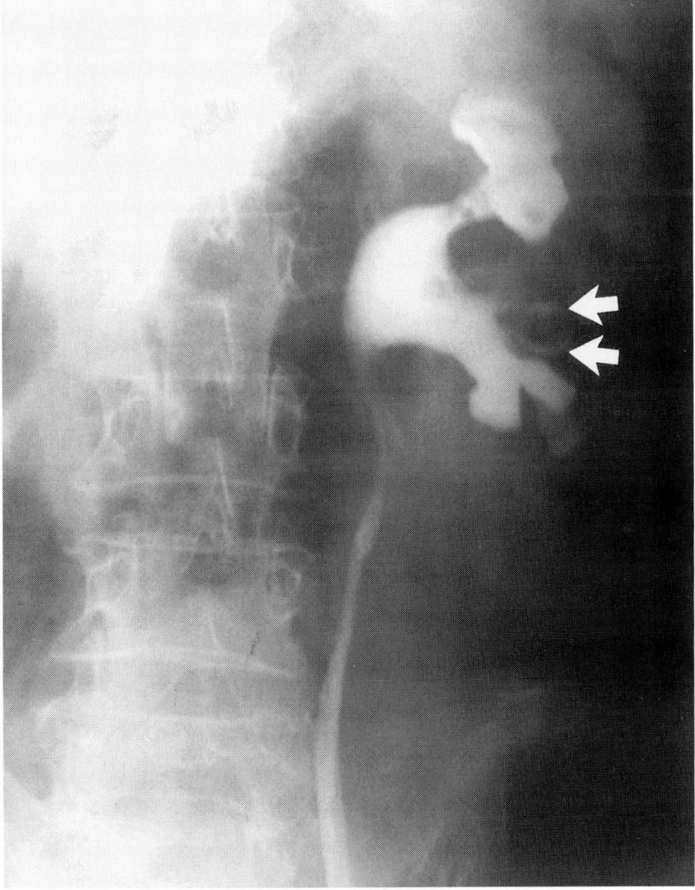

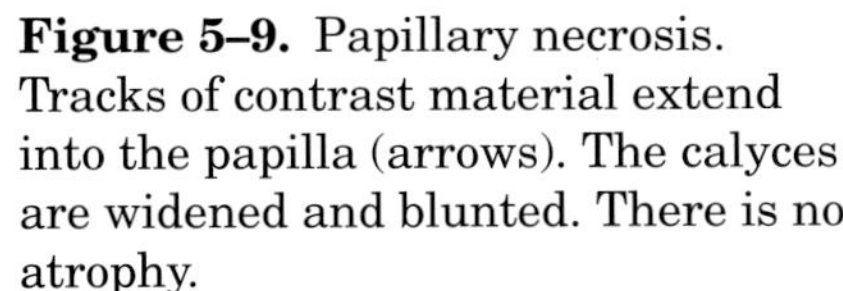
Figure 5–9. Papillary necrosis. Tracks of contrast material extend into the papilla (arrows). The calyces are widened and blunted. There is no atrophy.

RETROPERITONEAL FIBROSIS

Retroperitoneal fibrosis consists of an extensive fibrotic tissue reaction in the retroperitoneum around the aorta. A number of diseases should be distinguished from retroperitoneal fibrosis, including retroperitoneal hemorrhage from aortic leaks and retroperitoneal malignancies such as Hodgkin's disease. Causes include methysergide toxicity in patients suffering migraine headaches, inflammatory bowel disease, and fibrous reactions due to previous surgery and/or radiation. This process occurs in middle-aged males more often than females. It may extend from the level of the renal vessels to the iliac crest. These patients may present with renal insufficiency and bilateral hydronephrosis.

At intravenous urography, there is commonly hydronephrosis of one or both kidneys. The hydronephrosis is typically asymmetric. The ureters are often narrowed (Fig. 5–10*A*). This narrowing may be focal or may involve a long segment. Medial displace-

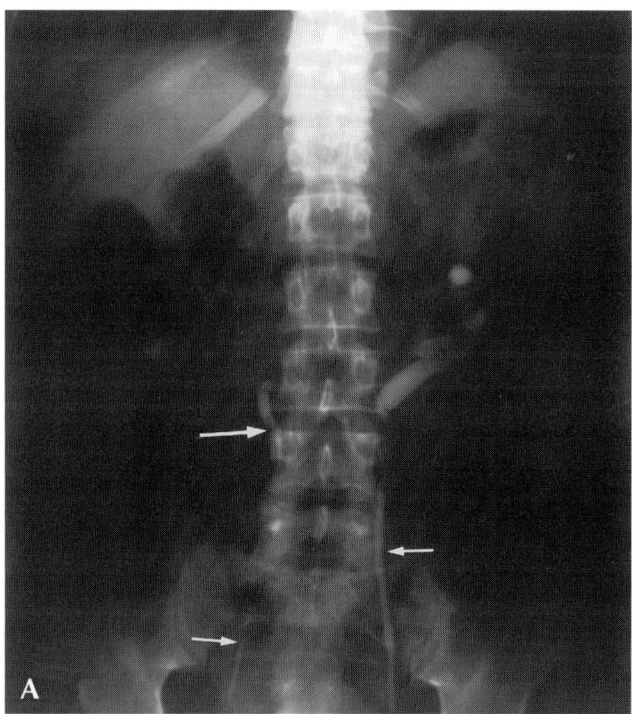

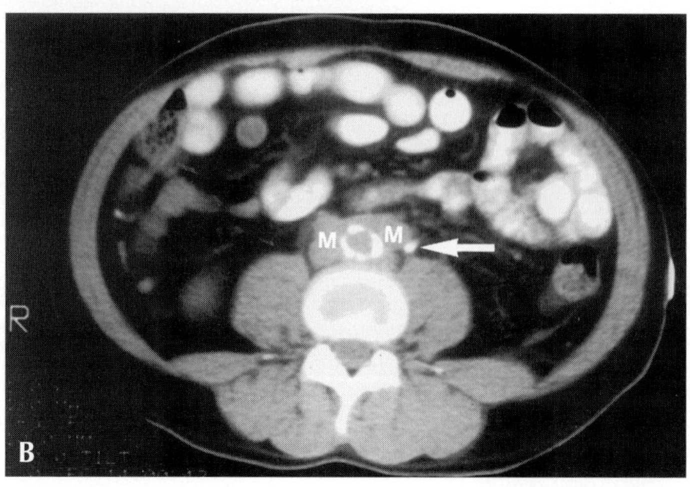

Figure 5–10. A. Retroperitoneal fibrosis. The ureters are deviated medially and narrowed (arrows). **B.** CT shows a soft tissue mass encasing the aorta (M). The left ureter is partially encased (arrow). The right ureter is not opacified and is somewhere in the soft tissue mass.

ment of the ureters may occur and is an important radiographic sign. This displacement can draw the ureters medially to a location over the spine, a finding commonly identified at the time of retrograde pyelography or antegrade pyelography.

Computed tomography will show hydronephrosis, but also shows a soft tissue mass in the retroperitoneum encasing the aorta, inferior vena cava, and ureters (Fig. 5–10*B*). Contrast enhancement may occur, but the mass may also be nonenhancing. At ultrasound, a poorly marginated hypoechoic mass will be seen in the retroperitoneum with associated hydronephrosis. The process may be very difficult to appreciate at ultrasound. On MRI this retroperitoneal mass typically will be of intermediate signal intensity on a T2-weighted image. This is in distinction to most malignancies, which are typically of high signal intensity on a T2-weighted image.

PYELITIS CYSTICA AND URETERITIS CYSTICA

Pyelitis cystica and ureteritis cystica consist of small cysts in the wall of the renal pelvis and ureter, respectively. These present as filling defects at the time of intravenous urography (Fig. 5–11). The cysts and filling defects are usually a few millimeters in diameter. They are thought to form from cells of uroepithelium that have penetrated downward from the mucosal surface. These cells ultimately become isolated from the surface and form fluid-filled cysts. Ureteritis cystica is seen more commonly in older women and may occur in association with *E. coli* urinary tract infection. In some patients, the lesions will regress after treatment of an underlying urinary tract infection. The most common location is in the proximal ureter.

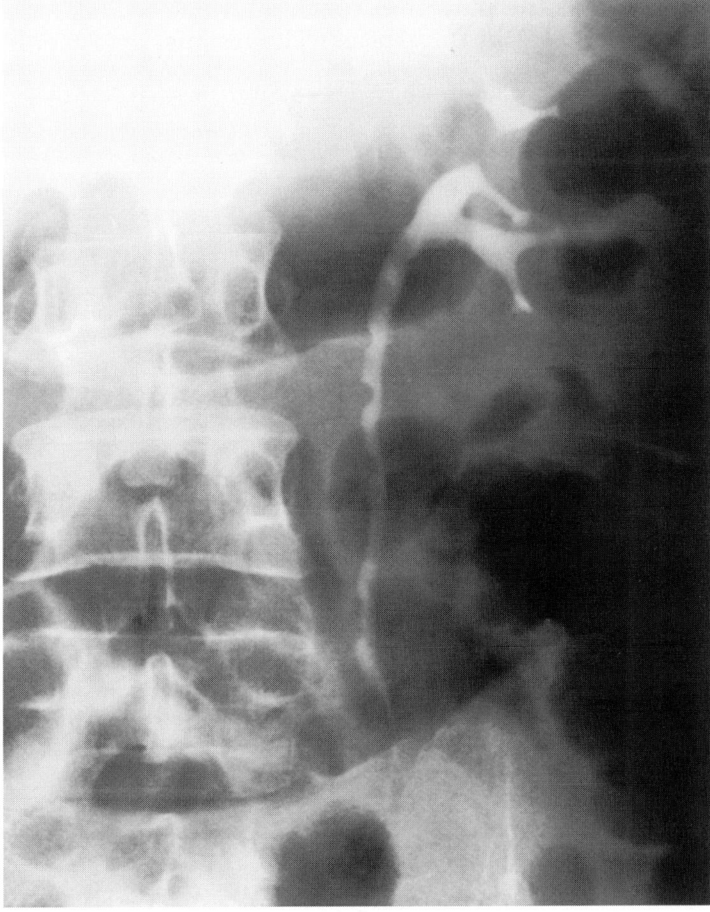

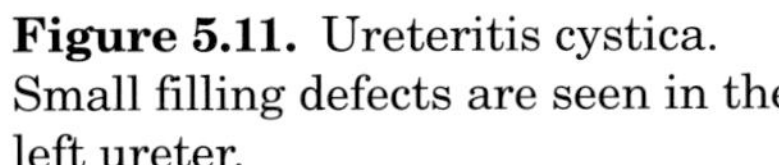

Figure 5.11. Ureteritis cystica. Small filling defects are seen in the left ureter.

MALACOPLAKIA

Malacoplakia is an inflammatory process involving the ureter. It is associated with a chronic urinary tract infection such as that produced by *E. coli*. Classically, the lesion is composed of submucosal nodules due to granulomas. These granulomas form as a consequence of defective lysosomal lysis of bacteria. Microscopically, inflammatory cells contain cat's eye inclusions, known as Michaelis-Gutmann bodies, which are pathognomonic of the disease. These are probably incompletely digested bacilli (usually *E. coli*). Malacoplakia is most common within the bladder, but also affects the ureters and the upper tracts. It is more common in women in the fifth and sixth decades. At urography, irregular filling defects are present. There may or may not be obstruction. Ultimately, strictures may develop. Most cases have multifocal masses. About half are bilateral and one-fourth are unifocal. These lesions may extend into the perirenal space and may lead to renal vein thrombosis. The lesions tend to be less rounded compared to ureticis cystica and more often cause dilatation of the ureter.

LEUKOPLAKIA

Leukoplakia is another inflammatory condition of the ureter. It usually involves the proximal one-third of the ureter, but there is frequently extension into the renal pelvis. It also occurs in the bladder. A urinary tract infection is usually present. However, the urinary tract infection may not be necessary for the development of this condition. This is a precursor of squamous cell carcinoma. Males are as affected as females. It is common in middle age. Hematuria may be present, and many of these patients will give a history of passing white chalky material in the urine. This is thought to represent epithelium. At urography there will be irregular filling defects in the ureters and renal pelvis. Many of these patients will have coexistent renal stones.

Chapter

6

Upper Tract Trauma

RENAL TRAUMA

Either blunt or penetrating trauma may injure the kidneys. However, the kidneys are relatively well protected under the rib cage by the musculature of the paraspinous and iliopsoas muscles. Cases of minor trauma that cause hematuria should raise concerns about other preexisting renal pathology. Clinical signs of significant renal injury include shock, hematuria, and flank ecchymoses. A high percentage of blunt injuries may be managed conservatively, but penetrating injuries are usually explored. Multiple classification schemes have been used for renal trauma. One scheme is as follows:

I. Contusion and superficial cortical injury.
II. Deep cortical injury.
III. Renal disruption with devitalized fragments and pedicle injury.
IV. Ureteral pelvic junction avulsion.

Injuries are more common on the left. Children are more easily injured because the kidneys are larger in relation to the size of the body; they also more often have a preexisting pathology. The mortality in patients with renal injuries is more often due to associated injuries than to the renal injuries.

For blunt trauma, patients should be evaluated radiographically if they have a history of gross hematuria or microhematuria associated with hypotension documented at any point, including in the field. All penetrating trauma should be evaluated radiographically.

Radiographic Findings

On a plain film of the abdomen, pedicle fractures, loss of the psoas shadows, or loss of the renal cortical outline may be suggestive of renal injury. Whether an intravenous urogram or a CT scan should be performed for the evaluation of the kidney in renal trauma is controversial. An intravenous urogram has traditionally been used and is felt by many to be adequate for evaluation of renal trauma. It is readily available and may be done rapidly with only a single radiograph after injection of intravenous contrast in the emergency room. This study will show whether the kidneys are functioning but may give little other information. CT scans, however, have the advantages of increased sensitivity and more accurate staging of the renal injury. Further, a CT scan may detect injuries to associated viscera. The advantages of CT are so great that we rarely perform intravenous urography in the trauma setting. CT should be performed using both oral and IV contrast material. Angiograms are rarely used at the current time. Angiograms may occasionally be useful in situations of pedicle trauma versus contusion or where vascular injury is suspected (see Chapter 7).

A Grade 1 injury (contusion and superficial laceration) may have a normal radiographic appearance, or there may be a decrease in function. At times there may be a heterogeneous appearance with a striated nephrogram. There may also be thinning of the calyces, which can be described as wispy in appearance. There is no urinary extravasation. Sometimes a superficial laceration may be identified on a CT scan. Small amounts of subcapsular blood or fluid may be seen.

A Grade 2 (deep cortical laceration) injury is identified when there is an area of low density extending in a linear fashion through the kidney and into the region of the hilum. This is the hematoma from a fracture, and it most often occurs between vascular branches. Fragments may be widely separated. There may also be small amounts of extravasation of contrast and perinephric blood (Fig. 6–1).

A Grade 3 injury (complete disruption or pedicle injury) will represent a catastrophic renal injury. On CT scan, these injuries will have large areas of devitalized tissue (Fig. 6–2*A*). Failure of a fragment of soft tissue to enhance implies that there is no blood flow.

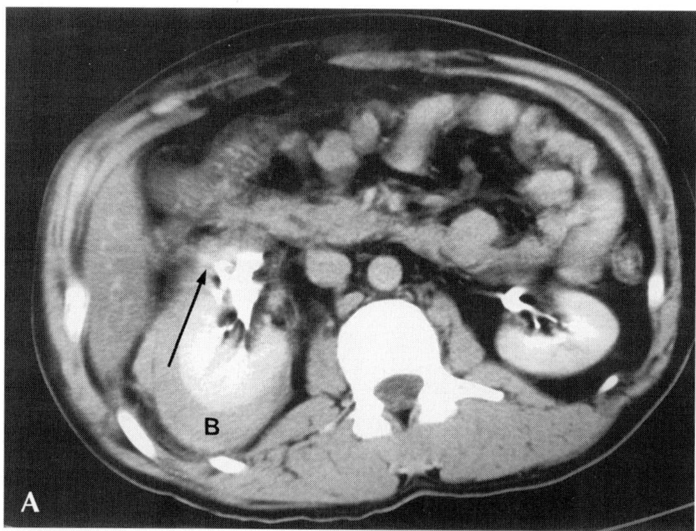

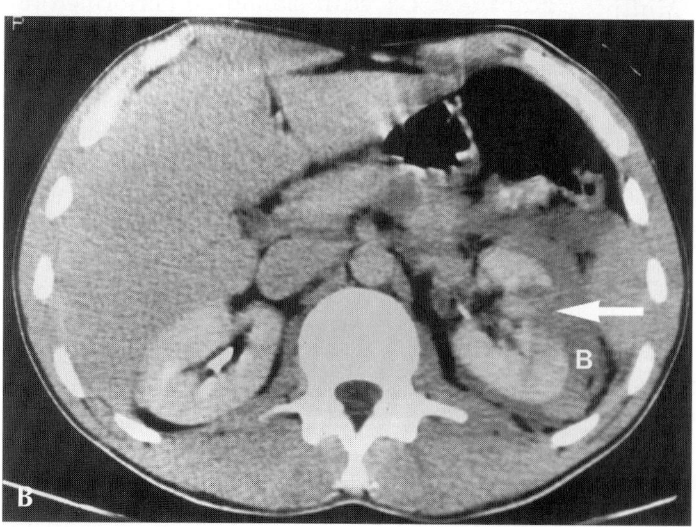

Figure 6–1. A. Perirenal blood (B). This CT scan was done with intravenous contrast material. This is a Grade 2 injury because small amounts of contrast material extravasation were seen (arrow). **B.** Another patient with a Grade 2 injury. A fracture (arrow) extends through the left kidney, and there is perirenal blood (B).

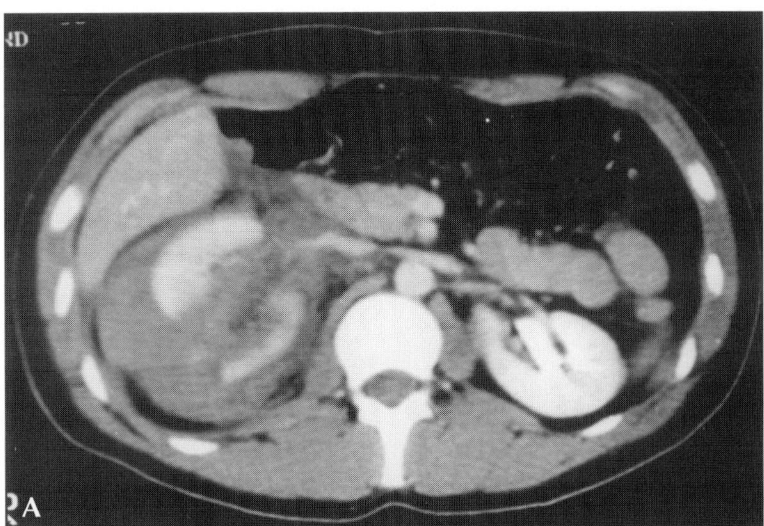

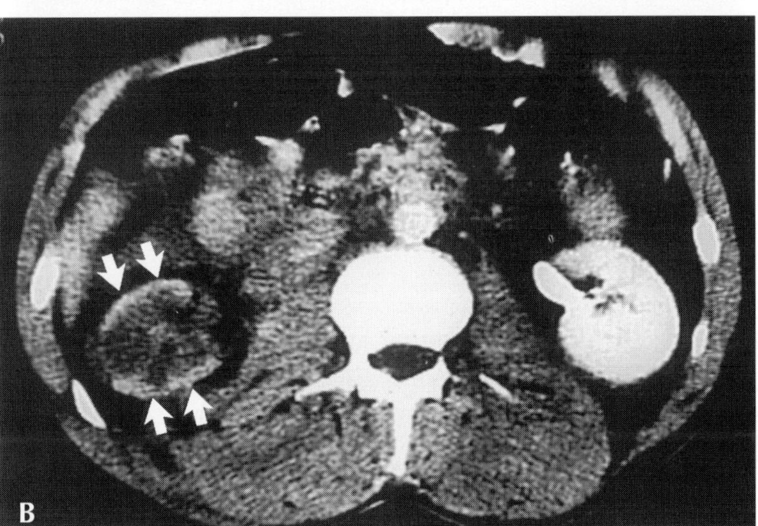

Figure 6–2. A. A Grade 3 injury of the right kidney. A large area of devitalized tissue in the central portion of the kidney is apparent. There is also a large perirenal hematoma. **B.** Vascular trauma with peripheral rim enhancement.

Peripheral rim enhancement of the otherwise nonfunctioning kidney or renal segment is seen as a consequence of vascular trauma (Fig. 6–2*B*). This is due to perfusion of the superficial cortex by capsular arteries. If the artery is avulsed, retrograde flow into the renal vein may be identified at CT. There may be large amounts of contrast material extravasation and hemorrhage.

A Grade 4 injury (ureteral pelvic junction disruption) should be suspected when there is extravasation of contrast material medial to the kidney (Fig. 6–3). In this situation, retrograde urography should be considered. This type of injury is often associated with either a penetrating trauma or a major deceleration injury.

Contusion of the Kidney

Contusion of the kidney (Grade 1 injury) is a relatively minor traumatic renal injury. Consensus today indicates that conservative nonoperative management is the best treatment. On intravenous urography this is manifest as an area of decreased enhancement. On CT an area of decreased enhancement with blurring of the renal border and blood or edema in the perirenal fat may be seen. Subcapsular collections of fluid and/or blood may be seen. These are usually crescent shaped and may compress the kidney. There may be focal swelling associated with contusion itself. At times, there may be prolonged and intense

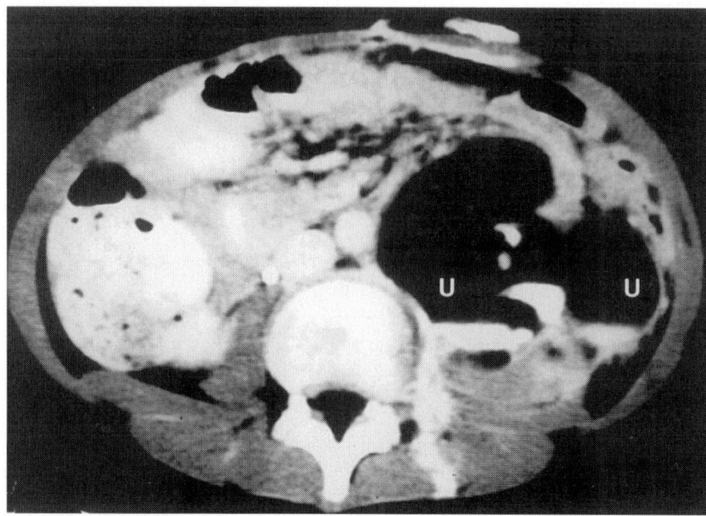

Figure 6–3. A ureteral injury with disruption of the ureteropelvic junction has occurred as a result of a gunshot wound. A gas-fluid level is present in the large left-sided urinoma (U).

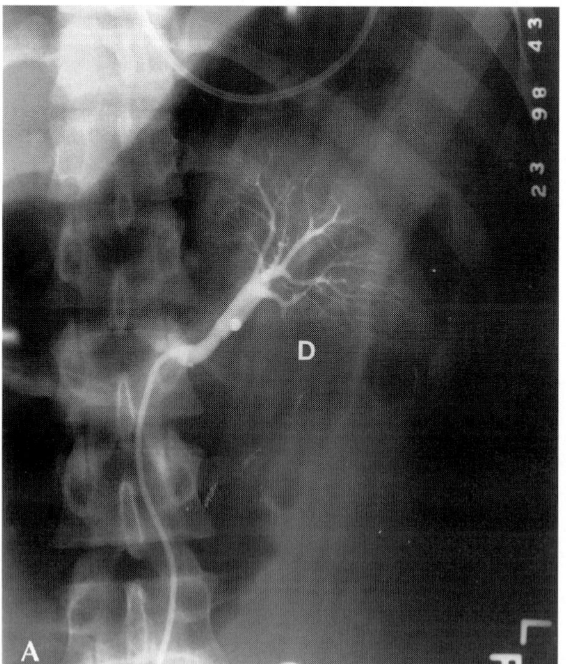

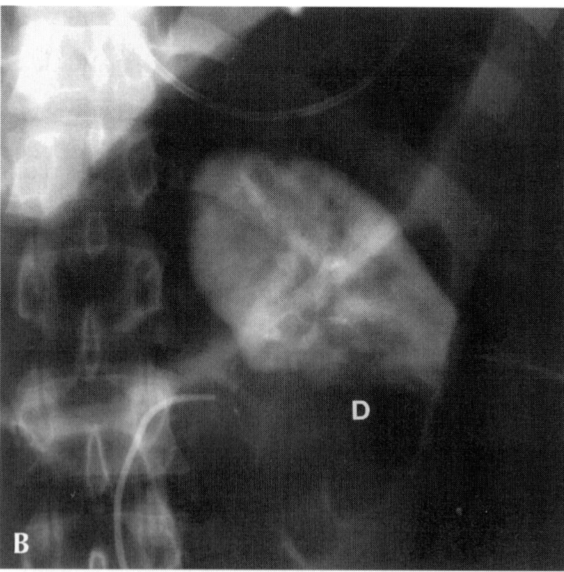

Figure 6–4. Two images from an angiogram of the left kidney after trauma. **A.** The early image shows flow to the upper pole but no flow to a devascularized lower pole (D). **B.** An image obtained several seconds later shows good enhancement of the upper pole but no contrast in the devascularized lower pole (D).

enhancement of the contused area as opposed to decreased enhancement.

Segmental Infarct of the Kidney

Trauma to the kidney may at times result in an infarct of a segmental area. This presumably is a result of contusion, with ultimate thrombosis of segmental blood vessels. On intravenous urography, computed tomography, and angiography this will appear as a wedge-shaped area of nonenhancement (Fig. 6–4).

Vascular Disruption

Vascular disruption (Grade 3 injury) may occur as a result of trauma. The artery is injured more often than the vein. Vascular pedicle injuries show a lack of enhancement on an intravenous urogram. Delayed films may show some faint cortical enhancement secondary to capsular arteries. Similarly, on CT there will be no enhancement of the kidney.

We currently perform CT in cases where vascular disruption is suspected. An abrupt cutoff of the renal artery just beyond its takeoff from the aorta will be visible. In the past, angiography was the mainstay in the evaluation of suspected vascular injury (Fig. 6–5). However, CT has largely replaced it. The CT scan can also exclude congenitally absent kidneys, ectopic kidneys, or nonfunctioning kidneys secondary to some other disease as potential causes for radiographic nonvisualization of the kidney.

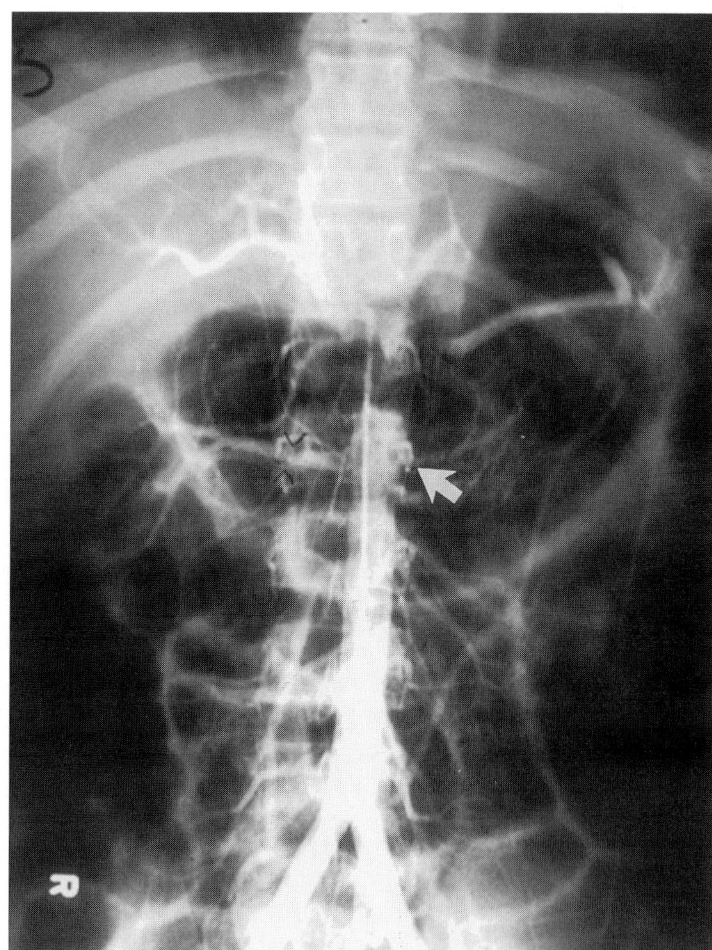

Figure 6–5. Abrupt cutoff of the left renal artery, indicating avulsion.

Ureteropelvic Junction Disruption

Ureteropelvic junction disruption (Grade 4 injury) is a serious sequela of trauma that is manifested by extravasation of opacified urine. This injury is more common in penetrating trauma. It is very unusual for the kidney not to be simultaneously injured. Therefore, there will usually be major abnormalities in the kidney. This is usually an indication for operative repair.

While the diagnosis may be seen at urography, CT is more sensitive to identify medial extravasation of contrast material (Fig. 6–3). It may be necessary to perform retrograde urography to confirm the diagnosis.

Chapter

7

Vascular Abnormalities

RENAL ARTERY STENOSIS

In the 1930s Harry Goldblatt demonstrated that decreased renal perfusion led to hypertension and that this process could be reversed. Renovascular hypertension is responsible for 2 to 4 percent of all cases of hypertension. Most renovascular hypertension is the result of atherosclerotic disease in the first few centimeters of the main renal artery (Fig. 7–1). Arteriosclerotic renovascular disease occurs most often in older age males. A second group of patients have renovascular hypotension due to fibromuscular dysplasia (FMD). This has been subcategorized into intimal, medial, or adventitial types. The intimal type is more common in children and occurs in the mid-renal artery away from the aorta. Medial dysplasia accounts for about 95 percent of the cases. It is most common in women between 20 and 50 years of age (Fig. 7–2). In the adventitial type, collagen surrounds the adventia, producing stenosis.

Many imaging procedures have been utilized for the diagnosis of renal artery stenosis. The gold standard remains arteriography. The superior resolution of this procedure, coupled with the ability to treat the lesion simultaneously via angioplasty, makes this the definitive procedure. However, angiography has the disadvantage of being invasive. Angiography can be performed using digital subtraction angiography (DSA). A small 4F catheter is placed in the vena cava or right atrium. After injection of a small amount of contrast material, the image before injection is subtracted from an image obtained after the injection of contrast. Only those structures containing contrast material (i.e., vessels) will be visible after this subtraction. DSA may also be performed after placing a catheter in the aorta and injecting both renal arteries. This digital technique has the advantage of rapid viewing of the image and an accuracy near that of traditional cut-film angiography.

The screening test of choice currently is captopril renal scintigraphy (Fig. 7–3). Captopril is an angiotensin-converting enzyme (ACE) inhibitor. Kidneys with significant renal artery stenosis (RAS) have increased production of angiotensin II, which leads to efferent arteriolar vasoconstriction. Increased pressure in the glomerulus allows continued normal filtration. Captopril inhibits angiotensin II production, causing efferent arteriolar dilatation. A resultant drop in perfusion pressure results in

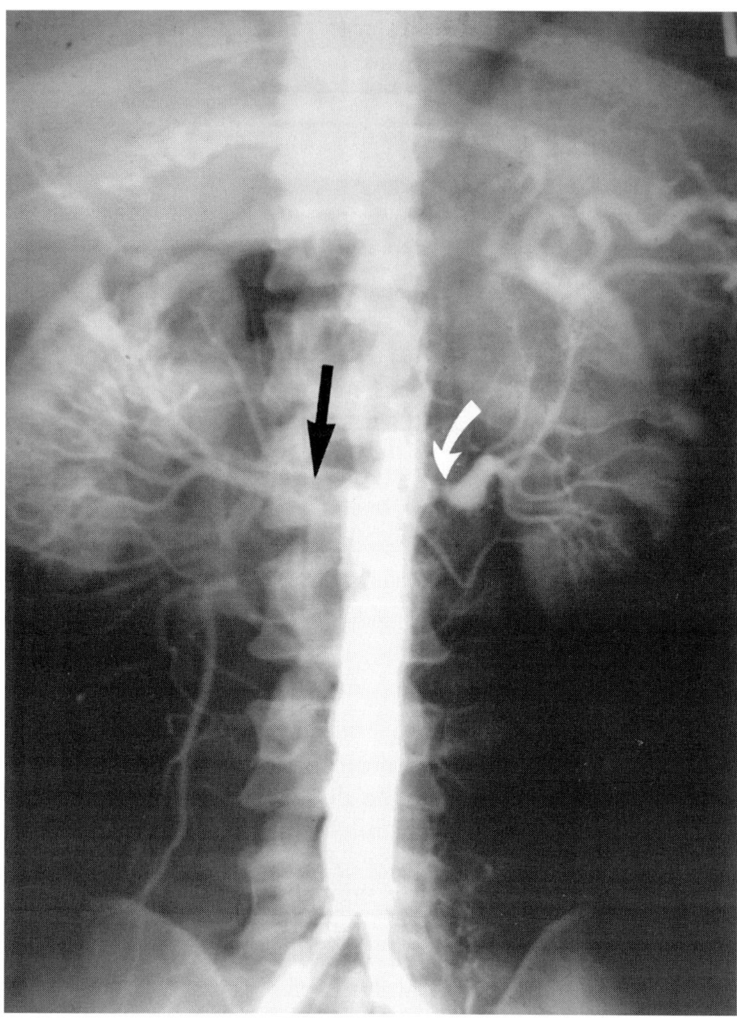

Figure 7–1. Bilateral renal artery stenosis. Severe stenosis of the right renal artery (straight arrows) is difficult to see because the artery overlies the vertebral body. The left renal artery stenosis is easier to identify (curved arrow).

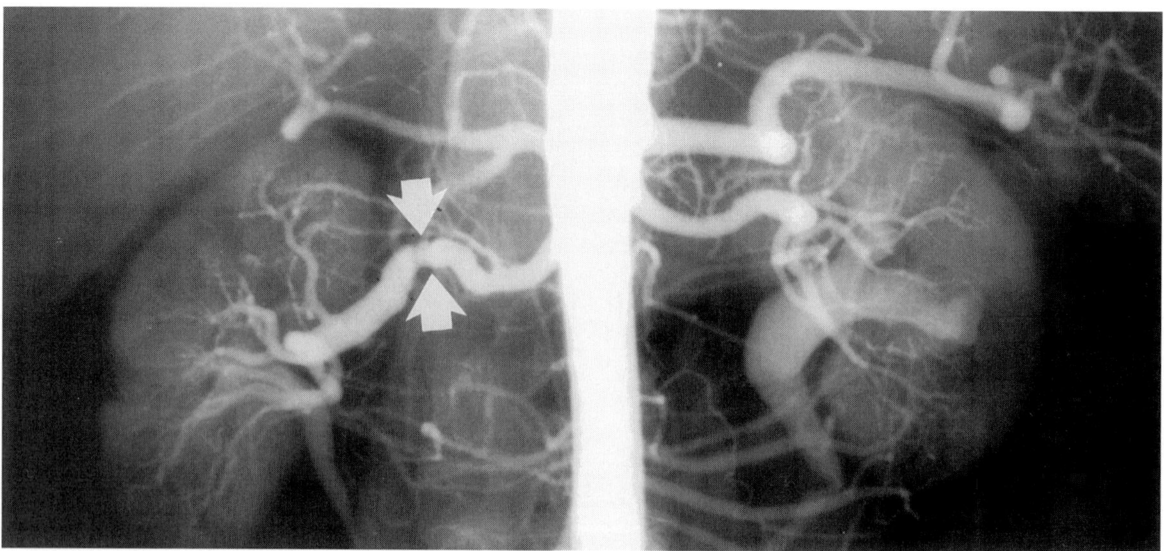

Figure 7–2. Fibromuscular dysplasia of the right renal artery (arrow).

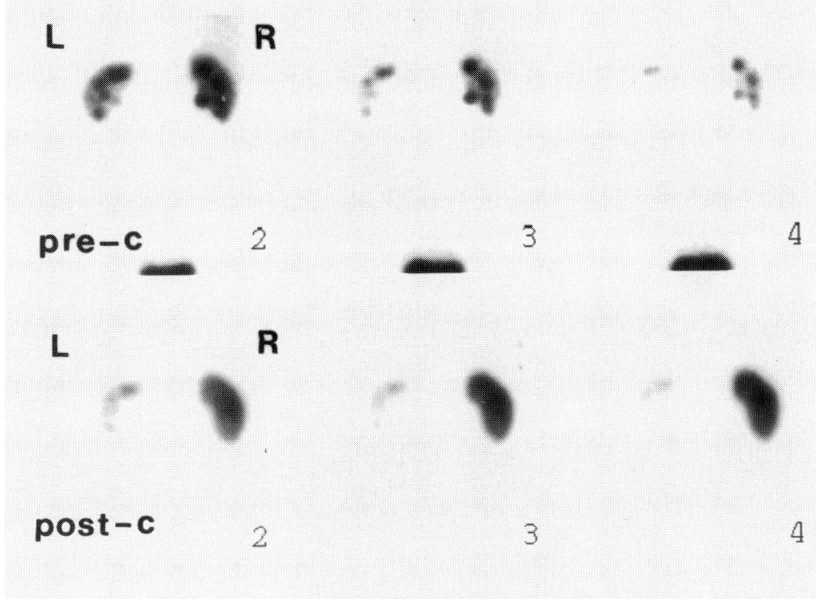

Figure 7–3. Captopril renogram, posterior images. The pre-Captopril images show a slight disparity between the two kidneys. After Captopril, perfusion to the left kidney is not maintained, indicating renal artery stenosis on the left.

decreased filtration in patients with significant RAS. This study is done by tracking and quantifying the excretion of technetium-99m/DTPA, iodine-131/iodohippurate, or technetium-99m. The abnormal kidney will have decreased uptake. Sensitivity for the test is about 80 to 85 percent, and specificity is 95 to 100 percent in patients with unilateral disease.

DOPPLER ULTRASOUND

This technique is not widely accepted because of difficulty in performing the exam. The main renal arteries are difficult to visualize even in the ideal patient. Up to 20 percent of patients have multiple renal arteries. This makes it impossible to be certain that all arteries have been fully examined. Doppler criteria for renal artery stenosis include a peak systolic velocity of 2 m/s in the stenotic zone and a peak systolic velocity in the stenotic zone that is 3.5 times the peak systolic velocity in the renal artery proximal to the stenosis or 3.5 times the peak systolic velocity in the adjacent aorta.

Interrogation of intrarenal vessels can be performed, and the resultant Doppler waveform can be analyzed. If a stenosis is present, these waveforms will be downstream from the stenosis and altered. A tardus-parvus waveform occurs. This is a waveform with a delayed upstroke and a time (from end diastole to peak systole) of greater than 0.08 seconds. In addition to difficulties in the performance of the exam, high sensitivities and specificities have not been widely reproducible. Therefore, this exam is not widely accepted.

MAGNETIC RESONANCE ANGIOGRAPHY (MRA)

This technique is still in the development phase (Fig. 7–4). It likely will be the test of choice in the near future. Magnetic resonance imaging techniques that cause blood

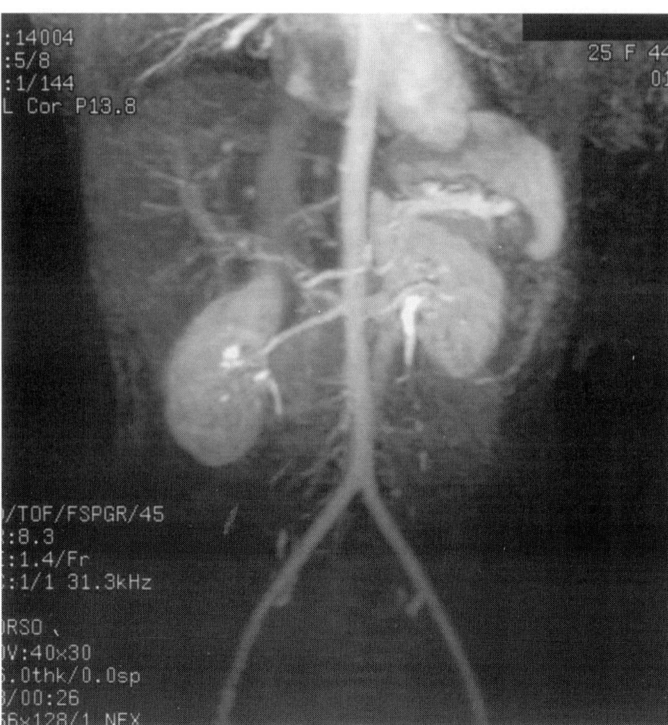

Figure 7–4. Magnetic resonance angiogram of the aorta and the renal arteries.

to appear white are utilized. These can be acquired over 10 to 15 minutes without iodinated contrast. Good results for detection of stenosis and for the detection of multiple renal arteries have been reported.

Currently, the MRA method of choice utilizes 40 mL of gadolinium DTPA contrast material by power injector at 1.5 mL/s. Three-dimensional gradient echo techniques are used while the patient holds his breath. This technique can be used in patients who have a creatinine level of less than 6.

COMPUTED TOMOGRAPHY ANGIOGRAPHY

Rapid volumetric abdominal data may be obtained using spiral CT while a power injector administers 150 mL of iodinated contrast. Angiographic images are then reconstructed. For living, related transplant donors, this computed tomography angiography (CTA) has replaced conventional angiography at many institutions. Currently, MRA is in use at more institutions than CTA for renal artery stenosis, although CTA has shown promise for stenosis detection in some series.

RENAL ARTERY ANEURYSM

Atherosclerotic renal artery aneurysms are usually calcified and present as spherical areas of calcification near the renal hilum (Fig. 7–5). They may be seen on plain films, urography, or computed tomography and are usually located in the proximal portion of the main renal artery, but can be located in more distal areas where the renal artery bifurcates. They are usually saccular aneurysms but may occasionally be fusiform. They may become partially filled with thrombus, and the thrombus may actually occlude the arterial lumen, leading to ischemia of portions of the kidney. Definitive diagnosis is best made at angiography.

At ultrasound, color Doppler may allow one to see flow within the mass. Vessels entering and exiting may also help to make the diagnosis. CT angiography may also be useful in evaluating this type of mass. Aneurysms of the renal artery may also

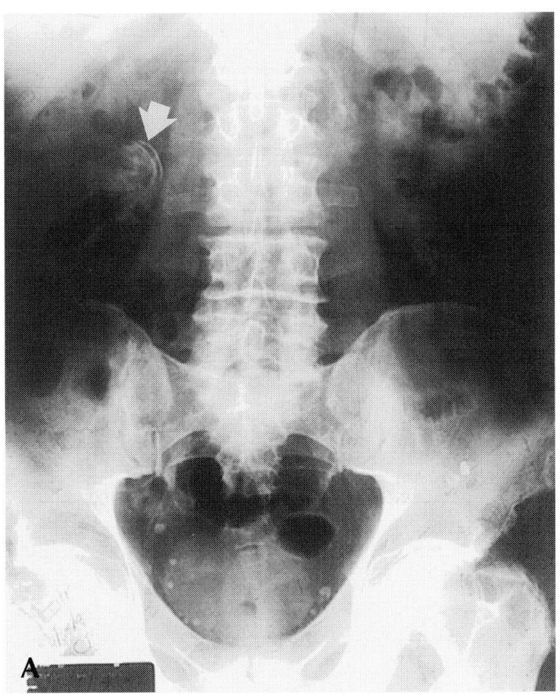

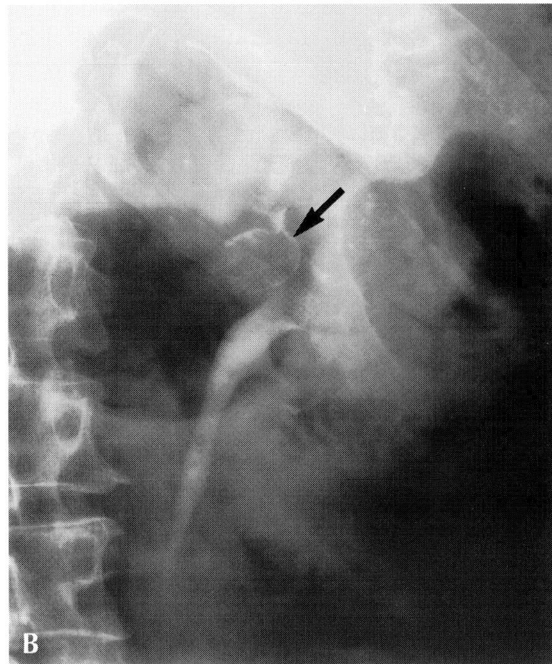

Figure 7–5. A. This plain film shows calcification of a right renal artery aneurysm (arrow). **B.** An intravenous urogram on a different patient shows a calcified renal artery aneurysm (arrow). **C.** Contrast-enhanced CT on another patient shows a left renal artery aneurysm (A) filled with thrombus. **D.** This angiogram shows contrast material filling a left segmental renal artery aneurysm (arrows). **E.** This digitally subtracted angiogram shows a renal artery aneurysm (arrow).

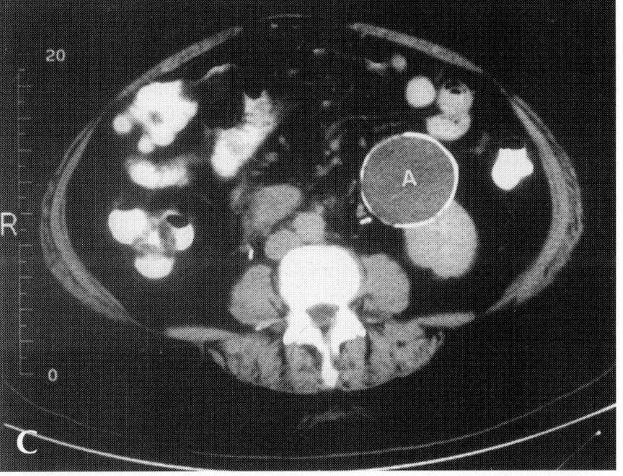

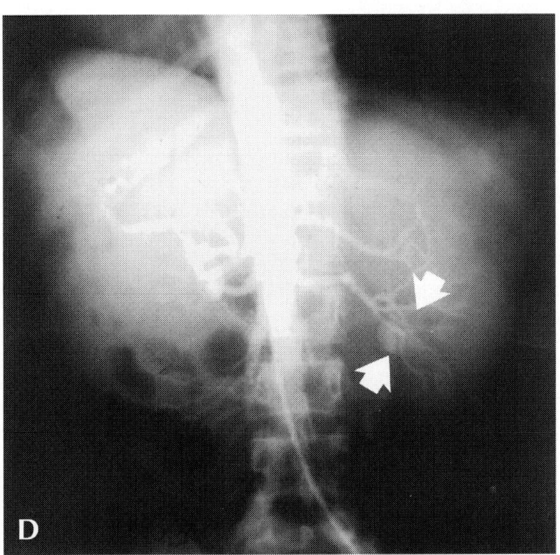

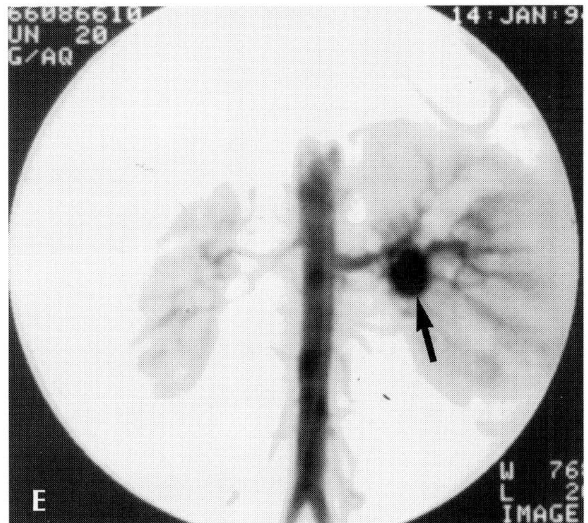

occur secondary to fibromuscular dysplasia, neurofibromatosis, or trauma, or on a congenital basis. Mycotic aneurysms may rarely occur. Distal intrarenal aneurysms occur with polyarteritis nodosa, IV drug abuse, vasculitis, trauma, and amphetamine abuse.

ARTERIOVENOUS MALFORMATION

Arteriovenous malformations (AVM) of the kidney are either congenital or acquired. The congenital type of arteriovenous malformation can be divided into two types: cirsoid or cavernous. The cavernous form is also called aneurysmal. The cirsoid type is the more common of the two and consists of multiple vessels coiled in a tight cluster. There may be more than one artery supplying this type of malformation. There may also be more than one draining vein. The malformation may cause hematuria. Cavernous malformations have a single large artery feeding a single dilated chamber that is drained by a single vein. AVMs commonly present in middle age and are more common in females. They may present with hematuria and are usually located in the medullary portion of the kidney.

The other type of arteriovenous malformation is one that is secondary to trauma. The trauma is usually penetrating trauma and today is most often the result of a renal biopsy (Fig. 7–6). In general, because there is no capillary bed, the arteries and veins feeding and draining either congenital or acquired malformations are large compared to normal arteries and veins. Clinically, patients may have an abdominal bruit and some may become hypertensive. This hypertension occurs because poor perfusion of the kidney distal to the shunt may cause secretion of renin. A pressure effect on the collecting system may also occur, leading to distortion of the calyces or even dilated calyces. Many of the small arteriovenous fistulae will heal spontaneously. These lesions are frequently followed if they occur after a renal biopsy.

At intravenous urography, a mass effect may be seen on the collecting system. Faint curvilinear calcifications may also be seen in the cavernous forms of these malformations. At CT, after the administration of contrast material, enhancement of the mass will be seen. At ultrasound, usually the AVM will present as an echogenic mass. The cavernous type may present as a hypoechoic mass. Color Doppler helps in determining that this is a vascular mass. At angiography, the mass will blush quickly,

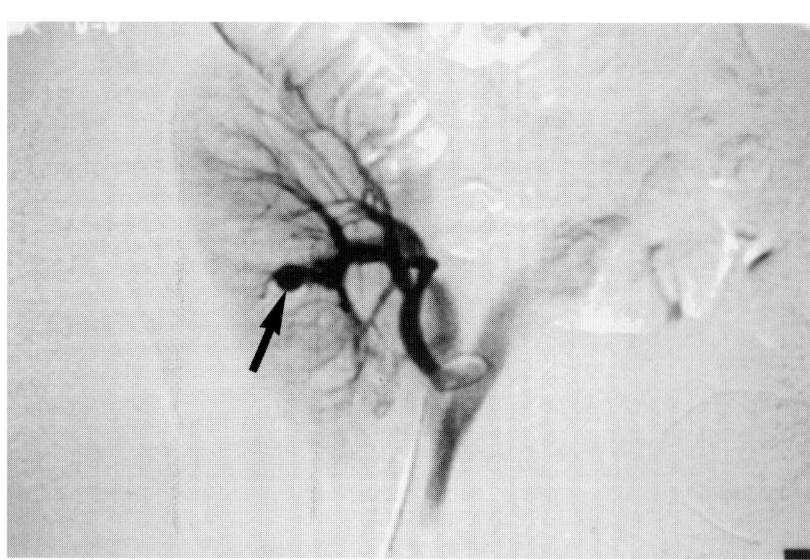

Figure 7–6. An angiogram of a renal transplant. An arteriovenous malformation secondary to biopsy is seen (arrow).

but early draining veins are not a prominent feature.

RENAL VEIN THROMBOSIS

Renal vein thrombosis may occur acutely or may be a more chronic process. When it occurs acutely, the result may be infarction of the kidney. When it occurs in a slower time frame, collateral vessels may develop while the kidney continues to function.

Renal vein thrombosis is common in the newborn and is usually associated with dehydration, frequently from diarrhea. Other causes of hypotension, such as dehydration and sepsis, may also cause renal vein thrombosis in newborns. The disease is more common in infants of diabetic mothers. In adults, renal vein thrombosis is usually due to an underlying kidney disorder, frequently the nephrotic syndrome or membranous glomerulonephritis. Occasionally masses may compress either the renal vein or the inferior vena cava, leading to thrombosis.

Renal vein thrombosis will produce a swollen engorged kidney because of the inability of blood to drain from the kidney. If the thrombosis is severe and acute without development of collaterals, arterial inflow to the kidney may cease and infarction may occur. At intravenous urography, the kidney affected will be larger and commonly will not enhance to the same degree as the other kidney. However, it will gradually accumulate contrast material over time and will show a delayed nephrogram. The appearance may be indistinguishable from that of complete, severe obstruction. Frequently, it will not be possible to see the collecting system well enough to tell if an obstruction is present or not. Ultrasound will usually show an enlarged, hypoechoic kidney. Because it is normally difficult to perform Doppler ultrasound of the renal vein, it may not be possible to directly image the clot in the renal vein. However, if Doppler ultrasound of the renal artery is performed and shows a high resistance pattern with reversal of diastolic flow, renal vein thrombosis should be suspected. Computed tomography may show an enlarged kidney that does not enhance as much as the other kidney. There may be little or no excretion of contrast material into the collecting system. Thin cuts (5 mm) may demonstrate a low-density thrombus in the renal vein. The gold standard for diagnosis of renal vein thrombosis remains renal venography. This is usually done by filming through the venous phase of a renal arteriogram. Currently, MRI is commonly used to visualize the renal veins. We use either cardiac-gated axial images or a magnetic resonance angiography sequence in an attempt to visualize the renal veins. Our preferred sequence is a three-dimensional phase contrast sequence after gadolinium.

POLYARTERITIS NODOSA

Polyarteritis nodosa is a subacute or chronic disease in which the walls of medium and small arteries become necrotic. This leads to stenosis or obstruction of the arteries and may lead to ischemia or infarction. Hypertension may also result. This may be an immune disorder, as it is commonly associated with infections in other areas of the body. The kidney may not be the only organ involved, because the heart, liver, and gastrointestinal tract are often affected. When the kidneys are involved, hematuria and protein loss can occur and the disease may even progress to infarction. Severe cases may lead to death. The diagnosis of renal involvement is usually made angiographically. Multiple small, approximately 2-mm, spherical aneurysms will be identified (Fig. 7–7). These aneurysms may heal as the underlying disease resolves or with treatment of the underlying infection. Even if aneurysms are not seen at angiography, there may be microscopic aneurysms in capillaries. These aneurysms may occasionally rupture and lead to a perinephric hematoma.

Patients with Wegener's granulomatosis, systemic lupus erythematosus (SLE), and scleroderma may also form intrarenal aneurysms. Wegener's patients have lung and/or airway involvement, manifested by

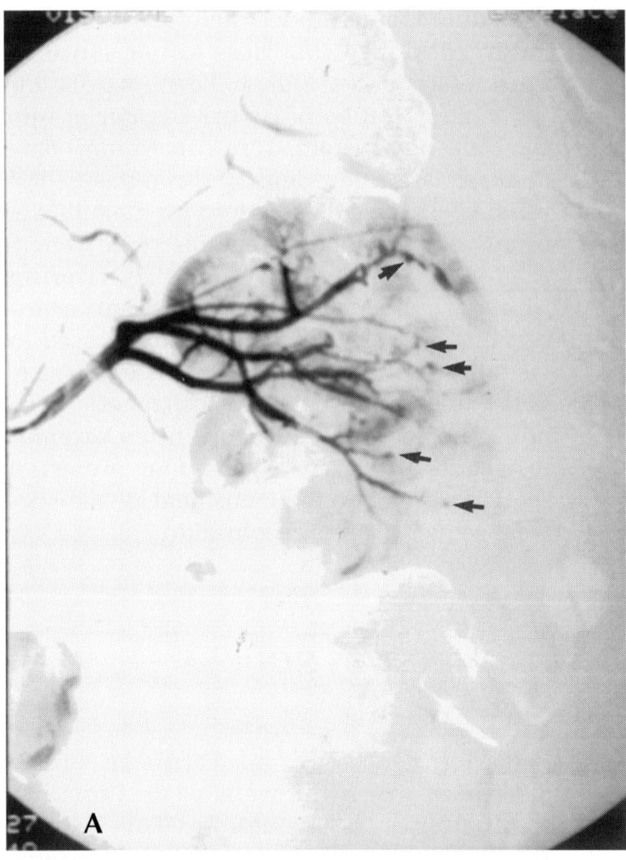

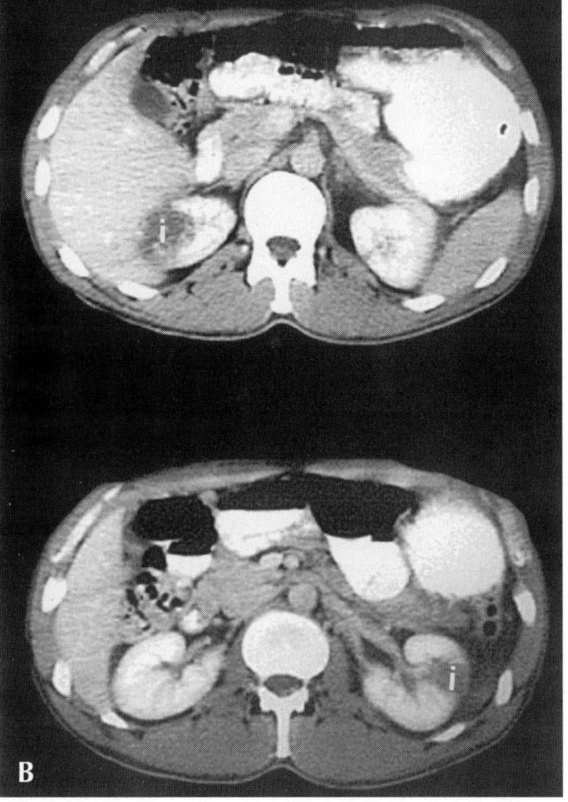

Figure 7–7. A. This angiogram of the left kidney shows numerous punctate aneurysms (arrows) in this patient with polyarteritis nodosa. **B.** CT in the same patient shows wedge-shaped peripheral low-density areas in both kidneys. These are areas of infarction (I).

necrotizing granulomas. The renal disease consists of a rapid glomerulonephritis with hematuria and proteinuria. SLE has small infarcts and microaneurysms. These patients develop a focal glomerulonephritis.

RENAL INFARCT/EMBOLUS

Emboli to the renal artery may result in infarction of either a portion of the kidney or the entire kidney if the main renal artery is occluded. The embolus usually comes from the heart. Atrial fibrillation and resultant thrombus formation in the atria or left ventricular aneurysm with resultant thrombus formation in the aneurysm may produce emboli. Bacterial endocarditis and rheumatic heart disease may also lead to the formation of emboli. Small emboli may come from the aorta in the form of cholesterol plaques. Patients with a renal embolus may present with acute flank pain, hematuria, nausea, vomiting, an elevated white blood cell count, and fever. Excretory urography will show absence of enhancement if the main renal artery is affected by an embolus, although there may be a few millimeters of enhancement around the periphery of the cortex via the capsular arteries. There is no excretion of contrast into the collecting system if the main renal artery is occluded. A cortical rim of enhancement, described earlier, is also seen on CT and is easier to appreciate using that imaging modality. If only small segmental areas are involved, wedge-shaped defects may be seen on CT and segments of decreased enhancement may be seen on excretory urography. Acutely, ultrasound will show an enlarged kidney with decreased echogenicity secondary to edema. Doppler will show decreased or absent arterial blood flow. Angiography will show an embolus or thrombus in the main renal artery when the kidney is involved. With segmental emboli, there is nonfilling of the arterial branches to a segment of the kidney.

Thrombosis of the main renal artery usually occurs as a result of severe narrowing from atherosclerosis. Thrombosis may also occur as a result of dissection due to trauma. The patient may be asymptomatic if the thrombosis occurs slowly over time. The kidney will be small unless occlusion occurs quickly. In that case, the kidney will be normal in size. The kidney will not enhance after IV contrast, although a small amount of peripheral enhancement may occur due to capsular arteries.

TRANSPLANT RENAL ARTERY STENOSIS

Stenosis of the arteries feeding a renal transplant may occur secondary to atherosclerotic disease in native vessels, faulty surgical anastomotic technique, reaction to surgical sutures, or vascular rejection. Various techniques have been used in an attempt to diagnose this problem noninvasively. Radionuclide renography has not been found to be sufficiently accurate. Doppler ultrasound has been utilized. The detection of a characteristic tardus-parvus waveform distal to a significant stenosis has been said to be diagnostic. This waveform involves measurement from the end of diastole to the first systolic peak. When this is longer than approximately 0.08 seconds, there is a delayed acceleration time or delayed upstroke, which suggests a stenosis proximal to the location where the Doppler measurement was been obtained. How accurate this finding is is still controversial. Stenosis of 50 percent will produce an angle-corrected peak velocity greater than 2 m/s in the stenotic zone with associated turbulent flow. The gold standard for evaluation for renal artery stenosis in a transplant is the angiogram. Angiography will clearly show the area of stenosis (Fig. 7–8). Transplant stenosis is treated with percutaneous transluminal angioplasty or surgical revision.

VASCULAR TRAUMA

Vascular trauma may occur secondary to abdominal trauma. The kidney is the organ

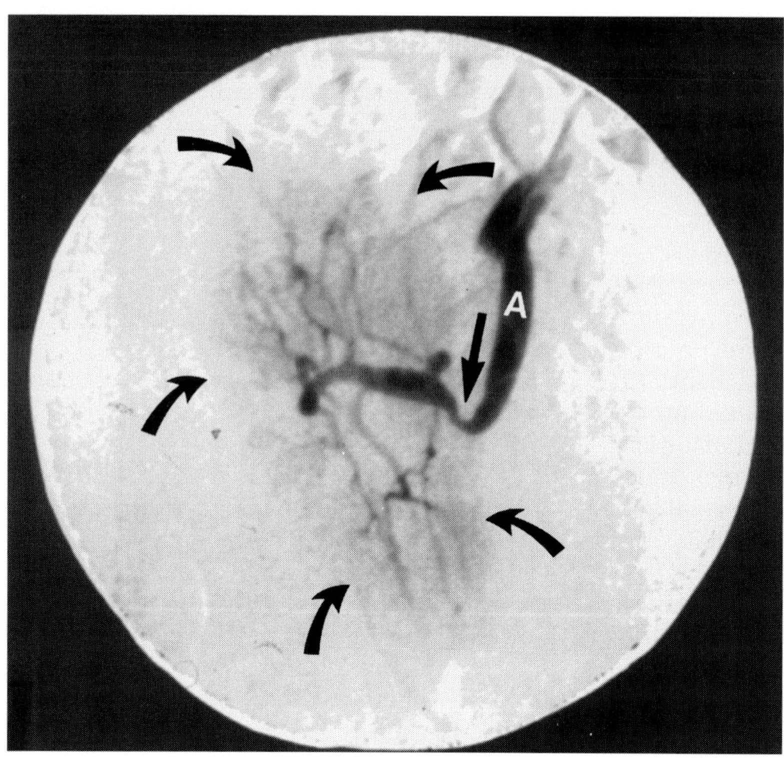

Figure 7–8. The right renal transplant is outlined by curved arrows. The straight arrow shows stenosis of the transplanted renal artery near the anastamosis with the iliac artery (A).

most commonly injured. If the main renal artery is avulsed, there is likely to be no enhancement or function of the kidney on excretory urography, computed tomography, or angiography. Because of some small cortical vessels that remain patent, at CT, the kidney may demonstrate a "rim sign" (see Fig. 6–2*B*) that, in the setting of renal trauma, is pathognomonic of pedicle injury. When an injury to the renal pedicle occurs with avulsion of the renal artery, there are frequently major injuries to adjacent organs and bones. However, an absent nephrogram may occur for reasons other than a renal pedicle injury and may be due to something as simple as overlying stool or bowel gas. Therefore, an absent nephrogram on IVP alone is not a sufficient reason for immediate surgery.

At renal angiography, a pedicle injury is indicated by an abrupt cutoff of the renal artery just beyond its takeoff from the aorta. Usually the avulsion is incomplete and the occlusion is secondary to injury to the intima of the artery.

RENAL CORTICAL NECROSIS

Renal cortical necrosis is an unusual condition in which ischemia of the renal cortex leads to necrosis of a portion of the kidney. A few millimeters of the most superficial cortex may be spared, presumably because of perfusion by capsular arteries. A few millimeters of cortex may also be spared in the juxtamedullary area, presumably because of perfusion by vessels from the medullary portion of the kidney. This condition sometimes results in complete death of all cortical tissue, but more often occurs in a patchy distribution. Most cases occur in association with pregnancy secondary to placenta previa, abruptio placenta, or septic abortion. Young children who are suffering from dehydration and fever are also at risk. Transfusion reactions, low cardiac output, and snakebite have all been implicated as causative factors. The condition may occur because of ischemia secondary to vasospasm of selected cortical vessels.

Acutely, the radiographic findings are those of diffusely enlarged kidneys. Accumulation of intravenous contrast material will be decreased, although there may be obvious enhancement of a few millimeters of superficial cortex and a few millimeters of inner cortex in the juxtamedullary position, which are still perfused. The presentation may simply be that of patchy cortical opacification. Over weeks or months the necrotic cortex calcifies and the parenchyma atrophies. The classic pattern is that of a line of calcification in the most superficial portion of the cortex and a line of calcification in the juxtamedullary position leading to a "tram-line" appearance. At CT, the contrast enhancement of the medulla and the superficial few millimeters of cortex can be seen with little or no enhancement of the necrotic cortex. Ultrasound may show a hypoechoic zone in the area of cortical necrosis. Over months the kidneys will shrink and be bilaterally small, smooth kidneys.

COLLATERAL VESSELS

Collateral arteries, veins, and varices may cause extrinsic impressions on the collecting system. These vessels may form in response to a major arterial stenosis or occlusion or venous thrombosis. Arteriovenous fistulas, vascular renal cell carcinomas, and congenital venous malformations such as a left-sided inferior vena cava may all lead to increased numbers and caliber of vessels around the kidney.

Chapter

8

The Bladder

NORMAL CYSTOGRAM

There are several clinical situations in which cystography may be indicated. Urinary tract infections in children raise suspicion of vesicoureteral reflux. A single infection in a male child indicates a need for a voiding cystouretherogram. Many physicians, however, allow two infections in a toilet-trained female child before performing a voiding cystourethrogram. There may be as much as a 50 percent incidence of abnormalities in children who are screened. In this clinical situation cystography alone is insufficient; voiding cystourethrography should be done. Some reflux may occur only during voiding. For that reason the catheter should be small enough that voiding can occur around it. The examination should be monitored fluoroscopically. In the normal patient, the voiding cystourethrogram will show complete emptying of the bladder without evidence of reflux in either the ureter or collecting system.

After trauma to the lower abdomen and/or pelvis, cystography is indicated to make certain that the bladder is intact. These patients often have pain or hematuria, and may have difficulty voiding. Examination of the bladder during the filling phase of an intravenous urogram is inadequate because the pressure within the bladder is insufficient to cause leaking even if the bladder is lacerated. Likewise, filling of the bladder after intravenous contrast for computerized axial tomography (CAT) scanning is inadequate to exclude a laceration. Retrograde cystography is necessary. A small percentage of lacerations may be missed using this technique unless the bladder is overfilled. The bladder should be filled with approximately 400 mL of contrast material or to the point of discomfort. At that time the bladder should be slightly overfilled with another 50 mL. Multiple films are obtained, and a postvoiding film is obtained to look for extravasated contrast material. It is important to use a relatively low concentration of iodinated contrast material so that bladder masses and injuries are not obscured by very dense material. Hematomas may cause displacement of the bladder or deformity of the walls of the bladder. Computed tomography cystography has been shown to be as accurate as traditional cystography when the bladder is filled retrograde before CT images are obtained.

NORMAL VOIDING CYSTOURETHROGRAM

A voiding cystourethrogram is similar to a cystogram in that the bladder is filled with dilute contrast material. The patient voids while being monitored by fluoroscopy. A video recording of bladder emptying may be obtained or 105-mm films of voiding may be obtained. The pressures become higher when the patient is voiding, and reflux will be more readily detected. Films should be taken of the kidneys and ureters during voiding. In addition, films of the bladder from the AP direction and both oblique directions should be obtained. Finally, images of the urethra should be obtained as the patient voids. If there is a concern about damage to the urethra, a retrograde urethrogram should be performed prior to passage of a catheter.

CALCIFICATION OF THE VAS DEFERENS

The vas deferens begins at the tail of the epididymis, passes within the spermatic cord, and enters the pelvis at the internal spermatic ring. It is closely applied to the lateral wall of the pelvis and makes a large arc to curve inferiorly and posteriorly. The vas deferens dilates as it approaches the excretory duct of the seminal vesicle. These two structures join to form the ejaculatory duct. On plain films of the pelvis, calcification of the vas deferens may commonly be seen. Usually only the portion of the vas deferens that is in the lower pelvis can be visualized when the vas deferens is calcified. This calcification is usually symmetric and bilateral, and appears as a beaded tube that is a few millimeters in diameter (Fig. 8–1). The calcification is common in diabetic

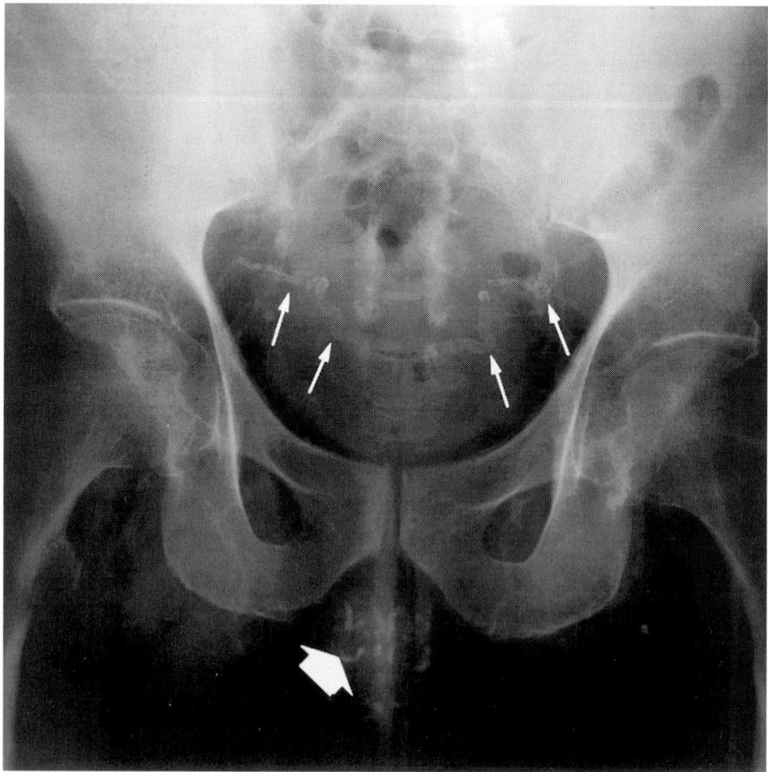

Figure 8–1. Calcification of the vas deferens (arrows). There is also penile calcification (large arrow).

males. It rarely occurs in nondiabetics. Calcification of the vas deferens has very little significance.

CONGENITAL ANOMALIES

Vesicoureteral Reflux

Vesicoureteral reflux occurs when the valve at the vesicoureteral junction does not function properly. The distal ureter angles into the muscular layer of the bladder wall via a tunnel under the epithelium of the bladder. When the bladder fills with urine, the urine acts to compress this tunnel and therefore occludes the distal ureter. This prevents reflux of urine into the ureters. In infancy, the course of the ureter in the tunnel is shorter and the bladder wall is thinner. Because of this, infants are more susceptible to vesicoureteral reflux. In infants and children, reflux will usually resolve with growth and maturation. Primary reflux is congenital and may have a hereditary component. It is more commonly unilateral than bilateral. Secondary reflux occurs when reflux occurs due to some other disease or acquired condition that affects the intramural tunnel at the ureterovesical junction. For instance, infants with myelomeningocele and neurogenic bladder may have high bladder pressures and can develop vesicoureteral reflux despite normal trigonal anatomy. This reflux may resolve with reduction of bladder pressure.

A diverticulum near the insertion of the ureter into the bladder may be associated with reflux. Infectious diseases, such as tuberculosis or schistosomiasis, may distort the trigone or scar the bladder so that reflux occurs. Patients with inflammatory bladder changes from radiation therapy to the pelvis may also develop vesicoureteral reflux.

Reflux is generally graded as follows: Grade 1, reflux into the ureter; Grade 2, reflux into the collecting system but no dilation (Fig. 8–2*A*); Grade 3, reflux in the collecting system with blunted forniceal angles (mild dilation); Grade 4, reflux in the collecting system with flattening of the papillae (moderate dilation); and Grade 5, reflux in the collecting system with convex calyces (severe dilation) (Fig. 8–2*B*).

Vesicoureteral reflux associated with infection may cause parenchymal scarring that may ultimately produce chronic renal disease (see Chapter 5). Initially the medullary pyramids are damaged by reflux, but ultimately cortical nephrons are affected, with resultant cortical thinning. Classically, reflux nephropathy has an appearance of focal renal parenchymal scarring and "clubbing" of associated calyces. This scarring tends to be worse at the upper and lower poles, possibly because of the shape of the papillae in these areas. These papillae tend to be more compound, and the collecting ducts are less oblique in their course. This has a tendency to allow reflux. Even if the reflux is surgically corrected, the parenchymal scar will not resolve, and radiographically the calyx may remain permanently clubbed. There is evidence that immature kidneys are more prone to the type of intrarenal influx into the periphery of the kidney and therefore are more prone to scarring. In general, it is felt that most scarring occurs in early childhood and that even if reflux occurs at a later age it is less likely to lead to scarring. It is unclear whether reflux of sterile urine will produce scarring.

The radiographic diagnosis of reflux nephropathy has long been made using a combination of intravenous urography and cystography. In the past, some advocated the use of intravenous urography as an initial step in determining if renal scarring was present. In the absence of scarring, no further workup is required. Others advocated cystography as a first step, arguing that a normal study precluded further evaluation. Currently, evaluation of a first urinary tract infection begins with a renal ultrasound. The ultrasound detects renal scarring but also may find evidence of hydronephrosis as well as other renal or bladder abnormalities, which may be causative. Following an ultrasound, voiding cystourethrography is performed to rule out reflux. At ultrasound the scars of reflux nephropathy are manifested by cortical thinning with areas of increased echogenic-

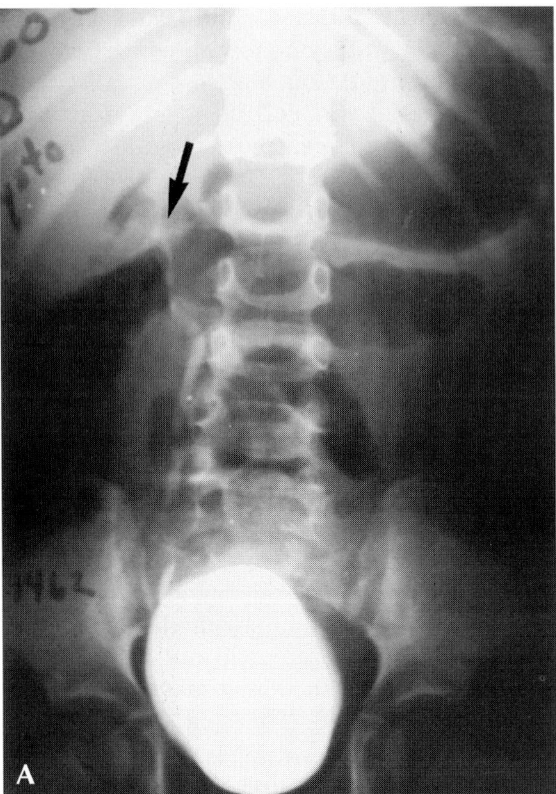

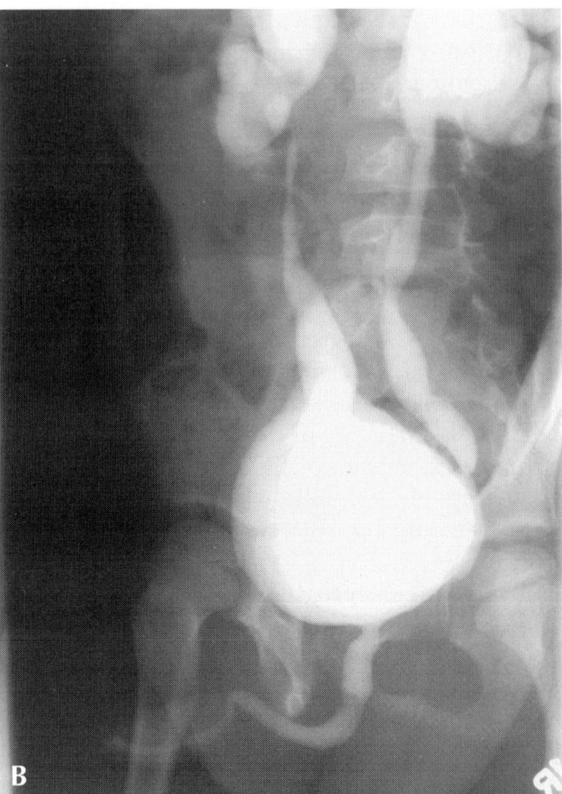

Figure 8–2. A. Grade 2 reflux on the right. Contrast material is seen in the right ureter and is faintly seen in the right renal pelvis (arrow). **B.** Grade 5 reflux bilaterally.

ity. However, reflux nephropathy can be distinguished from fetal lobulation by the regularity of fetal lobation and the fact that reflux nephropathy produces indentations that are irregular. In addition, no calyceal abnormalities are seen with fetal lobation. A differential diagnosis includes not only fetal lobation but also papillary necrosis, which may produce blunted calyces but usually will leave the parenchyma unscarred. Renal tuberculosis, which also may produce dilated irregular calyces and scarring, will usually have parenchymal calcifications. Finally, atrophy secondary to long-standing hydronephrosis usually causes more regular cortical thinning without focal scars.

Ectopic Ureter

The ureter may insert in the normal or orthotopic position on the bladder trigone or may insert in an ectopic site. Such ectopic insertion may be associated with ipsilateral ureteral duplication or ureterocele. In a completely duplicated system (with both orifices entering the bladder), the upper-pole orifice is usually located medially on the trigone, while the lower-pole orifice is formed more laterally. The lower-pole orifice is more likely to reflux because of a shorter intramural tunnel, while the upper-pole orifice is more likely to be located ectopically and to be obstructed. Ectopic sites of insertion in the male may include the bladder neck, prostatic urethra, or male genital ducts, including the seminal vesicle. In the female, the ureter may insert in the vagina, vaginal vestibule, uterus, or fallopian tube. Ectopia occurs much more commonly in females, and in males it is more often associated with a single nonduplicated system.

The clinical picture varies for males and females. Because ectopia in females commonly occurs distal to the bladder sphincter, the classical clinical presentation is one of constant dampness in a child who has been toilet trained and otherwise voids normally. Males, on the other hand, are more likely to present with urinary tract infections. However, both males and females not uncommonly present with infection.

Diagnosis by excretory urography (IVP) in part depends on the degree to which the upper-pole segment functions. Ectopia associated with a poorly functioning upper-pole segment and hydronephrosis may manifest as no function but show a "drooping lily" sign. This sign occurs because the lower-pole collecting system, which is usually missing an upper-pole calyx, is displaced inferiorly and laterally by a hydronephrotic upper-pole cap. In such instances, the insertion site of the distal ureter may not be visualized except through careful search for the ectopic orifice with retrograde injection of contrast. A finding of contralateral duplication with a single collecting system visualized on the affected side in a child presenting with infection should raise suspicion of ipsilateral duplication.

When the kidney parenchyma functions sufficiently to allow for visualization of the ureter, the actual ectopic insertion site may be visualized. In males, ectopic insertion into a seminal vesicle may be associated with poor renal function and a cystic dilatation of the seminal vesicle (see "Seminal Vesicle Cysts" in Chapter 9).

Since ultrasound is frequently the initial test of choice for evaluating urinary tract infection, there may be clues to ectopia identified on that study. In a nondilated system, separation of the renal sinus fat into two clumps should suggest the possibility of duplication. A hydronephrotic cap may be identified separate from the lower-pole ureter as a lucent cystic mass (Fig. 2–6*C*) with good through transmission. The ureter, usually dilated, may also be seen.

Cystography may reveal vesicoureteral reflux into the ipsilateral lower-pole segment. Ectopic ureters with insertion sites into the bladder neck or urethra may reflux as well. An ectopic ureter may or may not show radiographic evidence of an associated ureterocele.

Renal nuclear scanning is helpful to demonstrate ectopia by identifying a hydronephrotic cap as a scintigraphic "hole" or "cap." In children, for whom IVP is seldom the first radiographic exam, the nuclear scan may provide evidence for duplication by visualizing the ureters.

Ureteroceles (Cobra Head)

Ureteroceles are considered to be either orthotopic or ectopic. With an orthotopic ureterocele, the ureteral orifice is located at the normal position (Fig. 8–3). This is usually an incidental finding in an adult. Orthotopic ureteroceles are sometimes called simple ureteroceles. On the other hand, ectopic ureteroceles have an ectopic insertion of the ureteral orifice in the bladder. Ectopic ureteroceles are more often associated with a duplicated collecting system. The upper-pole moiety of a duplicated collecting system has a propensity to have an ectopic insertion. A ureterocele is a cystic dilatation of the intramural ureter.

Complications of ureteroceles include partial or complete obstruction and stone formation within the lumen of the ureterocele. Ureteroceles may become so large as to obstruct the contralateral ureteral orifice or may even cause bladder outlet obstruction. Ectopic ureteroceles may deform the bladder so that reflux occurs for the contralateral ureter. Radiographically on IVP, a ureterocele appears as a radiolucent filling defect that projects into the bladder. Urine in the ureterocele contains more dilute contrast than urine in the bladder. Because of this disparity, the wall of the ureterocele is clearly visualized (Fig. 2–8). For orthotopic ureterocele in adults, this creates a radiographic appearance that is usually referred to as a "cobra head." Lucent masses within the ureterocele lumen are usually secondary to stones. Ectopic ureteroceles may drain a portion of the kidney that functions poorly. These ureteroceles are larger and appear as a lucent mass in the bladder on intravenous urogram. At ultrasound a thin echogenic line in the bladder will usually be identified (Fig. 8–3). Because ureteroceles may cause a mass appearance in the bladder, the differential diagnosis often includes stones, blood clots, and bladder neoplasms.

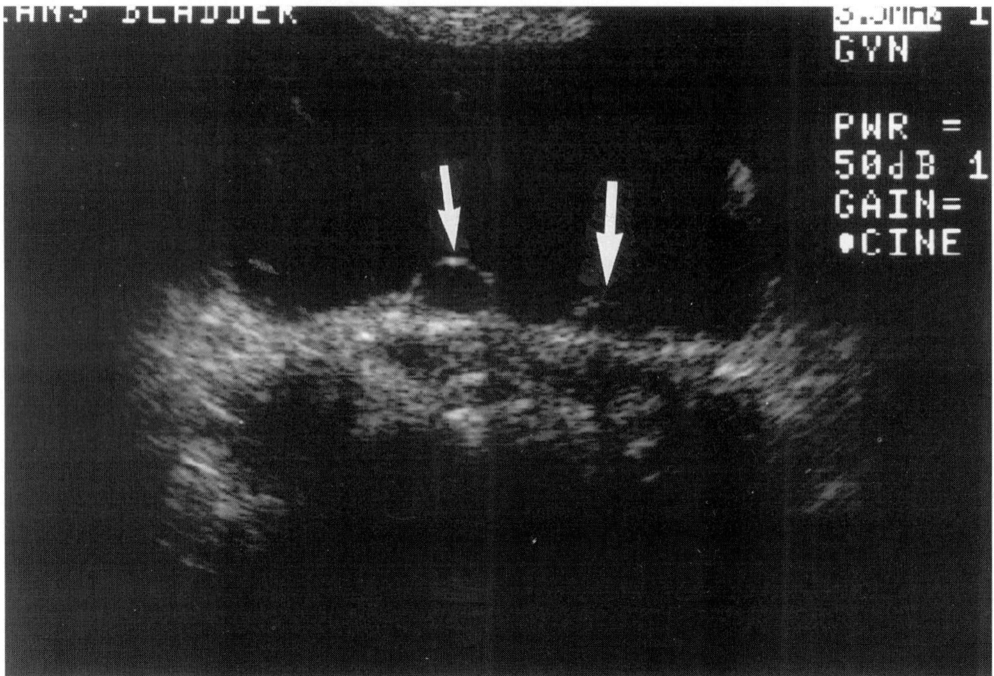

Figure 8–3. Bilateral orthotopic ureteroceles (arrows). A transverse ultrasound image of the bladder.

Eagle–Barrett Syndrome

Eagle–Barrett syndrome or prune-belly syndrome classically consists of the triad: absent abdominal musculature, bilaterally undescended testicles, and urinary tract abnormalities. The syndrome occurs only in males, although absence of abdominal musculature has been described in females. The urinary tract abnormalities involve the kidneys, ureters, bladder, and urethra. The kidneys may have renal dysplasia or hydronephrosis. Not uncommonly, the findings are asymmetric, and one kidney may be completely normal. The ureters are usually tortuous and dilated (Fig. 8–4). The dilatation is worse distally, and the ureters are also elongated. Obstruction is usually not present. Vesicouretero reflux is frequently present and massive. The ureters peristalse poorly, probably because of a patchy absence of muscle in the walls of the ureters. The muscle may be replaced with fibrous tissue. Likewise, the bladder may have areas of deficiency of smooth muscle. The bladder is often large, but is usually not trabeculated (Fig. 2–13). The prostatic urethra is frequently dilated, with tapering at the level of the membranous urethra and an appearance that may resemble posterior urethral valves. Prostatic hypoplasia is present and may be the cause of the dilated prosthetic urethra. The verumotatum is either small or absent. Cryptorchid testicles are present.

At birth, the diagnosis is frequently easily made because of the defect in the abdominal wall musculature. This defect affects the muscles of the lower abdominal wall worse than those of the upper abdomen. The defect may be asymmetric. The overlying skin and soft tissues have a wrinkled appearance suggestive of a prune. As children age, the wrinkling disappears and the children have a potbelly appearance. The cause of this syndrome has never been clear. It may occur secondary to the hydronephrosis and hydroureter in utero with resultant developmental failure of the abdominal wall musculature. Others feel that this syndrome results from a mesodermal abnormality.

Urachal anomalies, including a patent urachus and urachal cyst, are associated with prune-belly syndrome. A patent urachus occurs when the urachal pathway from

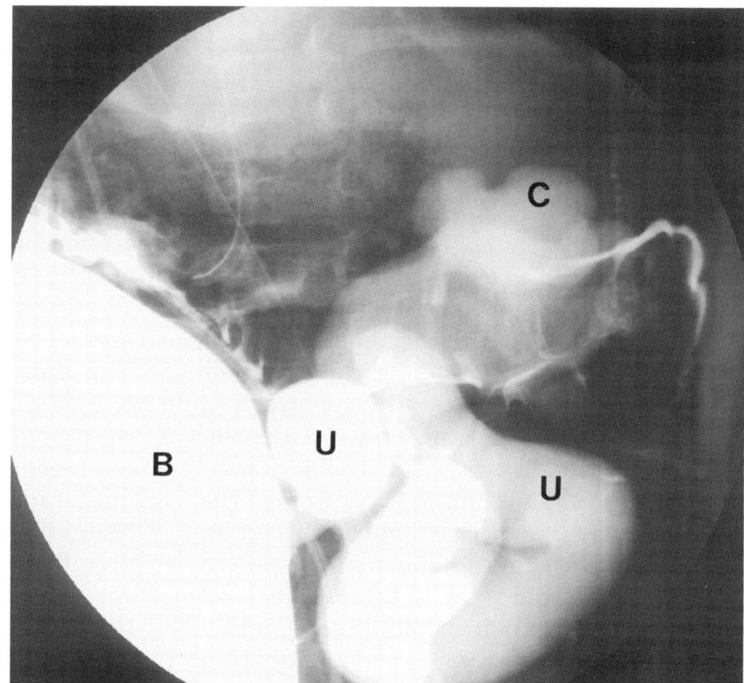

Figure 8–4. Prune-belly AP film shows the bladder (B), dilated left ureter (U), and dilated calyces (C) of the left kidney.

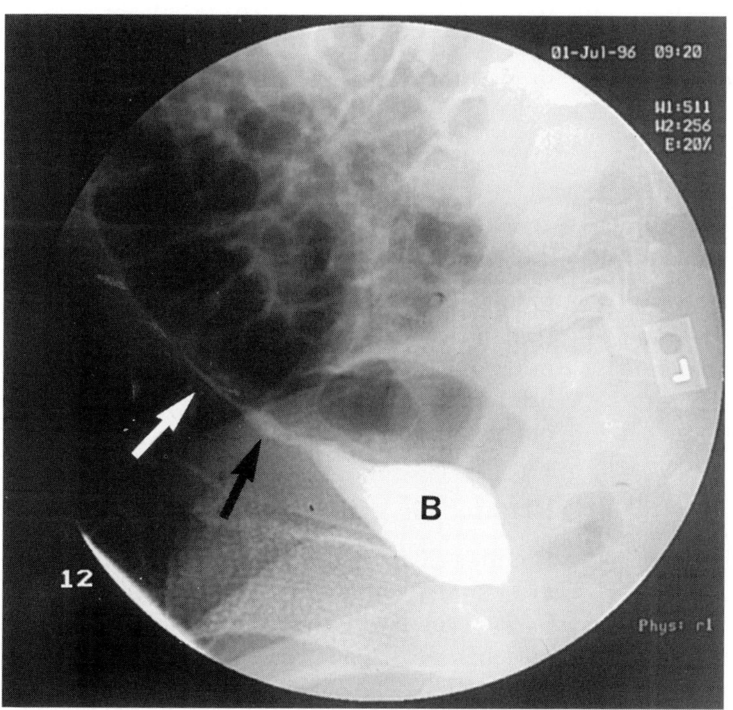

Figure 8–5. Patent urachus. A lateral film shows a line of contrast material (arrows) extending from the bladder (B) to the anterior abdominal wall.

the bladder to the umbilicus remains open (Fig. 8–5). This may cause urine to leak from the umbilicus. If the umbilical end of this pathway closes off, the remaining urachus forms a urachal cyst that is filled with urine and frequently becomes infected.

Myelomeningocele with Neurogenic Bladder

Normal bladder function depends on a closed urethra while the bladder is progressively distended. As the bladder nears capacity, brain stem centers receive impulses indicating the need to void. During voiding, the detrusor muscle contracts as a result of parasympathetic impulses from the sacral spinal cord. When the bladder contracts, the bladder neck forms a funnel and the sphincters around the urethra relax. The sacral micturition center lies between S2 and S4 and is connected to the bladder via a sacral reflex arc. In the past, neurogenic bladders have been classified as either upper or lower motor neuron bladders. The upper motor neuron bladder results when there is a lesion separating the brain stem control center from the sacral center. Lower motor neuron bladders are a result of separation of the bladder from the sacral micturition center. In general, the upper motor neuron type of bladder is referred to as hyperreflexive and the lower motor neuron bladder is called areflexive. However, simple classification does not always fit the clinical situation perfectly and lesions may cause overlap between these types of bladders.

Myelodysplasia is the most common cause of neurogenic bladder dysfunction in children. It occurs due to disruption of the posterior spinal elements, usually in a caudal location. A meningocele forms when only meninges extend beyond the confines of the spinal canal, while a myelomeningocele implies that neural tissue protrudes as well. In a lipomyelomeningocele, fatty tissue is associated with the neural elements as a protruding mass. The neurologic sequelae from myelodysplasia are variable and, unlike spinal cord trauma, do not produce a discrete "level."

With myelodysplasia the most common type of bladder is the upper motor neuron bladder or spastic bladder. This bladder is hyperreflexive. There may be lack of coordination between the bladder detrusor and urethral sphincter, causing bladder sphincter dyssynergia. Patients may not be able to perceive bladder filling or bladder emptying. Sphincter dyssynergia with voiding produces high bladder pressures that, when transmitted to the upper urinary tract, result in deterioration. The result is often upper tract dilatation seen on either urography or at ultrasound.

Obstruction of the distal ureters may occur secondary to the hypertrophied bladder wall. When voiding cystourethrography is performed, reflux may or may not be seen. The bladder will frequently be vertically oriented, and numerous trabeculations will be seen. This is sometimes referred to as a "Christmas-tree" bladder. If micturition is watched fluoroscopically, the sphincter may be seen to contract inappropriately. These patients may have reflux into the prostatic ducts leading to prostatic calculi. The anterior urethra will be poorly distended distal to the external sphincter, and there is usually incomplete emptying of the bladder. For patients with myelodysplasia and spinal cord injury patients, care must be taken when performing cystourethrography if the lesion is above approximately T5. Autonomic dysreflexia with diaphoresis, headache, severe hypertension, bradycardia, and even stroke may occur when the bladder is distended. In adults it may be possible to guard against autonomic dysreflexia in adults with a 10- to 20-mg dose of oral nifedipine (an alpha blocker) 30 minutes prior to the procedure.

Spina Bifida Occulta

Spina bifida occulta is a frequent incidental finding on plain films of the lumbar spine. This has no significance in terms of urologic abnormalities. In the past it was thought that people with spina bifida occulta were more prone to other abnormalities of the lumbar spine and more prone to back pain, but even this is now disputed.

Bladder Diverticula (Hutch-type)

Bladder diverticula in infants and children are usually congenital anomalies as opposed to the type of diverticula that occur in older patients, which are caused by bladder outlet obstruction. The congenital type of diverticulum is a result of herniation of bladder mucosa through muscular fibers of the bladder due to deficient development of the muscle in the bladder wall. This usually occurs slightly superior and lateral to the orifice of the ureter. A diverticulum in this location is often called a Hutch diverticulum (Fig. 8–6). These diverticula may deform the uretrovesi-

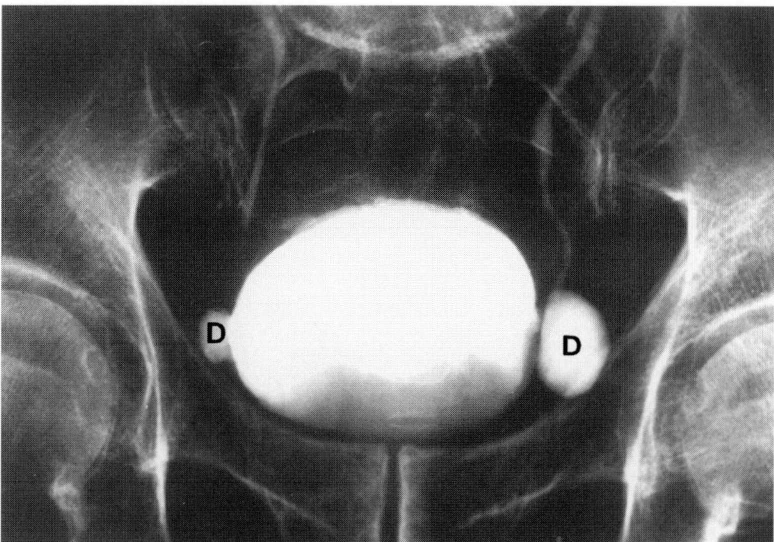

Figure 8–6. Bilateral bladder diverticula (D). These are Hutch-type diverticula.

cle junction and lead to either obstruction or reflux on a voiding cystourethrogram. The diverticula may also lead to stagnation of urine because of incomplete emptying. Whether or not this happens depends on the width of the neck of the diverticulum. Stones may also form within the diverticulum. Diverticula are rare causes of bladder outlet obstruction in infancy and children. Imaging of the diverticula may be difficult. It may be nearly impossible to confirm the diverticulum as a cause of obstruction. Multiple modalities may be used to image these diverticula, including cystography, voiding ureterography, ultrasound, and CT. Films should be taken after voiding to see if the diverticulum empties.

The Hutch type of bladder diverticulum must be distinguished from "bladder ears." These are transient protrusions of bladder down the inguinal canal in males. They usually have a wider neck than a diverticulum and resolve with aging.

Most other bladder diverticula occur in older patients, more often in males, due to bladder outlet obstruction. These often occur near the bladder base (Fig. 8–7), frequently anterolateral to the ureterovesical junction. These may become so large that they obstruct the bladder outlet. They may also become a site for the development of bladder cancer.

Sacral Agenesis

Sacral agenesis is part of a larger syndrome known as the caudal regression syndrome. Mal- or nondevelopment of the lower lumbar and sacral portions of the spinal column occur. Absence or poor development of the lower extremities may be evident. Sacral agenesis occurs in association with maternal diabetes, and there may be a genetic basis for this syndrome. Genitourinary (GU) and gastrointestinal (GI) anomalies including anal/rectum malformations and other anomalies of sex and pelvic organs may appear. Patients may present with bowel/bladder motor problems. Sacral agenesis is best appreciated on a lateral film of the pelvis, although it can be suspected on the basis of an AP film. This syndrome is more common in male infants than in female infants. The range of urologic abnormalities seen includes renal aplasia or dysplasia, neurogenic bladder, malformed external genitalia, anal atresia, and sirenomelia. Magnetic resonance imaging is useful in evaluating the distal spine and assessing the extent of abnormality.

Exstrophy/Epispadias Complex

Bladder exstrophy and epispadias of the penis are part of a spectrum of rare abnor-

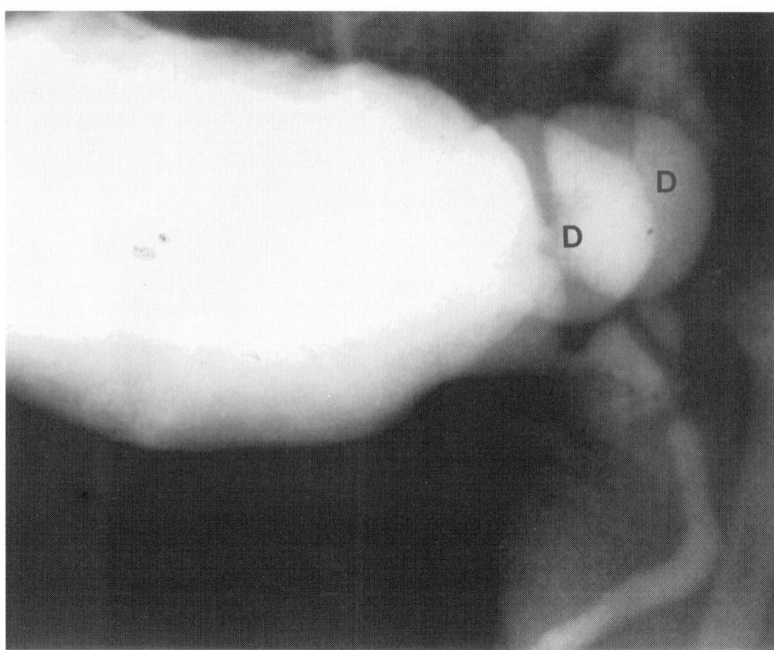

Figure 8–7. A voiding cystourethrogram, lateral film. Two diverticula (D) are present at the bladder base.

malities that occur as a result of failure of proper development of the anterior abdominal wall. Midline fusion of mesodermal tissue located below the umbilicus does not take place. Males make up approximately 75 percent of the cases of bladder exstrophy. The bladder may be open to the skin of the anterior abdominal wall. The bladder mucosa will be continuous with the skin. This bladder mucosa, which should have transitional cell origin, may become metaplastic. These patients are at an increased risk for adenocarcinoma of the bladder. If there is epispadias, then the urethral mucosa may cover the dorsum of an attenuated penis. The urethra opens on the dorsum of the penis. In the female the urethra is short, with widely separated labia and a cleaved clitoris. Kidneys and ureters are usually normal.

This anomaly should be suspected when a plain film of the pelvis shows pubic diastasis. The two pubic bones should be between 5 and 9 mm apart up to age 2, and between 4 and 8 mm between ages 2 and 13. If this distance is widened, approximately 65 percent of the patients will have exstrophy of the bladder and another 25 percent will have epispadias. The remaining 10 percent of the patients will have other syndromes involving the pelvis. The only other radiologic conditions accounting for pubic diastasis are pregnancy and pelvic trauma. In addition to widening of the pubic symphysis, the iliac bones are rotated outward, as are the pubic bones. The most caudad portions of the ureters sweep more laterally than usual and penetrate the bladder wall in a perpendicular course. The distal ureters may be dilated slightly. These patients may have associated ureteroceles and/or fibrosis at the ureterovesical junction leading to ureteral obstruction. Gastrointestinal and skeletal abnormalities may also occur.

TUMORS OF THE BLADDER

Rhabdomyosarcoma

There are four histologic types of rhabdomyosarcoma: embryonal, alveolar, pleomorphic, and sarcoma botryoides. Sarcoma botryoides has a grapelike appearance, which is very characteristic. In the bladder it usually occurs within the wall and grows into the lumen, sometimes obliterating the lumen. Rhabdomyosarcoma is the most common pediatric soft tissue sarcoma, and rhabdomyosarcoma of the GU tract is the most common form. Males are affected about twice as often as females. Rhabdomyosarcomas occur most often in the first 3 years of life and usually arise from near the trigone or bladder base. The tumor mass may protrude out of the urethra in females. A cystourethrogram will show a lobulated mass at the bladder base with thickening and irregularity of the bladder wall (Fig. 8–8*A*). The distal ureters may be obstructed. The tumor may also extend into the urethra. It may not be possible to tell if this tumor originates from the bladder, prostate gland, or vagina. Ultrasound and CT may help to stage these tumors. Rhabdomyosarcomas have mixed echogenicity or mixed density with an irregular and bulky appearance (Fig. 8–8*B,C*).

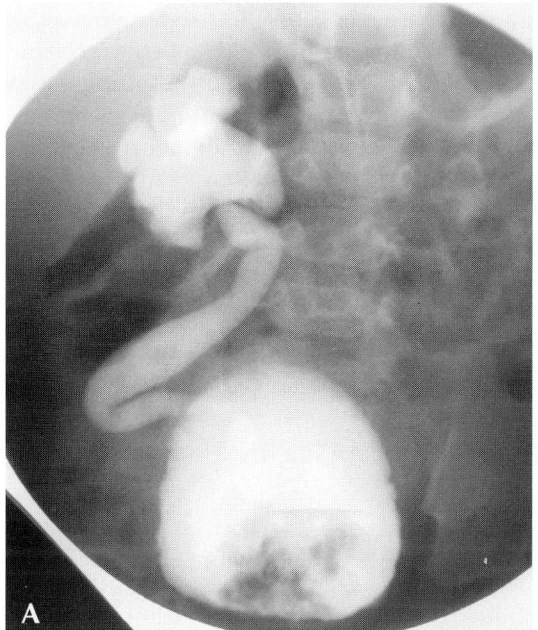

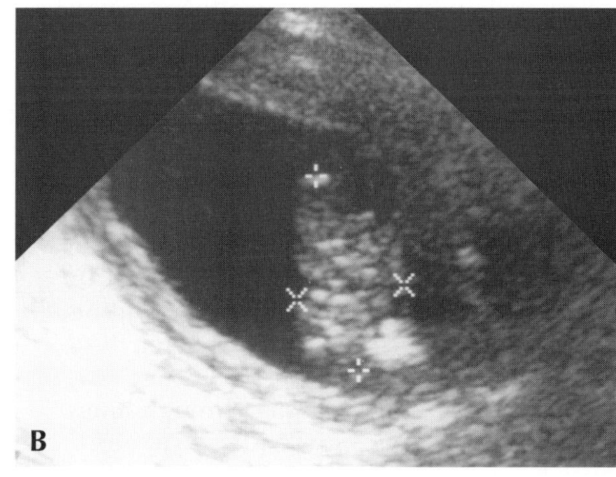

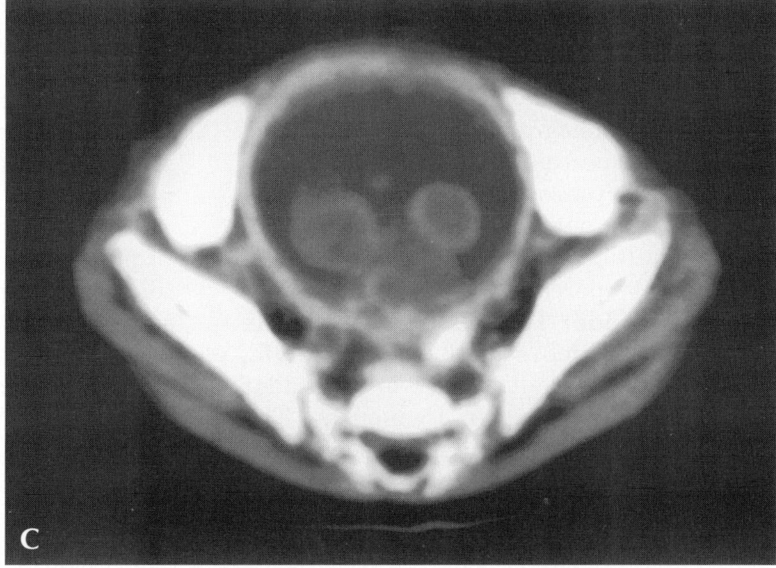

Figure 8–8. **A.** A cystogram in sarcoma botryoides. There is an irregular filling defect near the bladder base caused by the tumor. Reflux occurs into the obstructed right ureter. **B.** Sagittal ultrasound of the bladder in the same patient showing the tumor. **C.** CT shows a cluster of masses projecting from the posterior bladder wall.

Transitional Cell Carcinoma of the Bladder

Over 90 percent of bladder carcinomas are of the transitional cell variety. Squamous cell carcinoma and adenocarcinoma account for the remaining 10 percent. Approximately 80 percent of bladder tumors occur in males and they are much more common in elderly males. Multiple exogenous agents have been associated with transitional cell carcinoma. Almost all are aromatic amines. The most common of these is cigarette use. Cigarette smokers have an incidence that is two to five times higher than that of nonsmokers, and 30 to 40 percent of all bladder cancers are attributed to smoking. Aniline dye workers also have an increased risk. Numerous other workers who deal with chemicals also have an increased risk. Prior pelvic irradiation and phenacetin have also been associated with this tumor. *Schistosoma haematobium* has a strong association with bladder cancer. Jewett and Strong originated a bladder carcinoma staging system: Stage 0, mucosal; Stage A, mucosal lesion extending into submucosa; Stage B1, extension less than halfway through muscle; Stage B2, extension more than halfway through muscle; Stage C, tumor extending through muscle into perivesicle fat; Stage D, tumor through muscle and perivesicle fat with distant metastases.

Cellular grading of transitional cell carcinoma has also been performed. The cells may be graded as well differentiated (Grade 1), moderately differentiated (Grade 2), or poorly differentiated (Grade 3).

Plain film radiography usually is normal. Fewer than 1 percent of bladder tumors calcify. Excretory urography should be performed to rule out upper tract involvement because multicentric tumors are very common. Twenty percent of those with upper tract or bladder tumors have multiple tumors. For tumors of the renal pelvis, there is a 50 percent chance of a bladder tumor developing within 15 months. The intravenous urogram must be performed with good compression to detect the upper tract tumor. The sensitivity of excretory urography for the detection of bladder tumors is approximately 75 percent (Fig. 8–9*A*). Cystography is not significantly better. Ultrasound has been reported to detect more than 90 percent of bladder tumors if the bladder is adequately filled at the time of the exam. CT is useful in staging; it can be helpful in finding para-aortic or pelvic lymph nodes (Fig. 8–9*B*). It can rule in penetration of the bladder wall but is not adequate for staging a degree of bladder wall involvement.

Recently, MRI has been utilized in some centers to stage bladder cancer. Surface coils and endorectal coils have been used. Because of the neovascularization associated with cancer, there is greater enhancement of neoplastic tissue. Reported accuracies of MR for bladder cancer staging have ranged from 73 to 96 percent. These values are about 20 percent higher than those of CT. The best techniques currently involve using fast or ultrafast T1-weighted images plus intravenous gadolinium. MR is quite good at differentiating between muscular invasion and invasion of perivesicle fat.

PELVIC LIPOMATOSIS

Pelvic lipomatosis is the benign accumulation of fat in the pelvis and is usually seen in black middle-aged males, although cases may occur in other sexes and races. Patients may present with frequent dysuria, nocturia, and hesitancy. They may also have ureteral obstruction. Hematuria and urinary tract infections are occasionally seen. These males are frequently hypertensive. The cause of the fat accumulation is unknown.

Plain films of the pelvis show a striking radiolucency in the region of the bladder, secondary to the fat. Contrast studies show a bladder that is taller and narrower than usual. This has been described as teardrop-shaped or pear-shaped. The distal ureters are usually medially deviated. The middle portion of the ureter may be laterally deviated. Barium enema studies may show striping of the rectosigmoid colon. On ultrasound the pear shape of the bladder may sometimes be appreciated. On CT the abun-

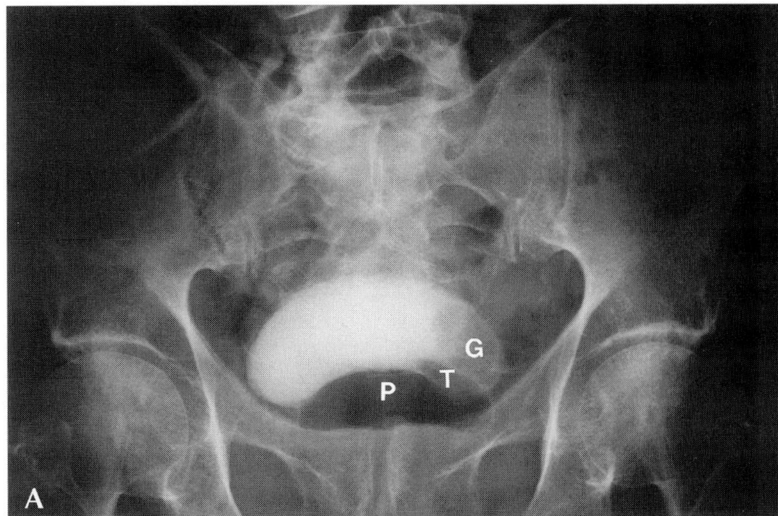

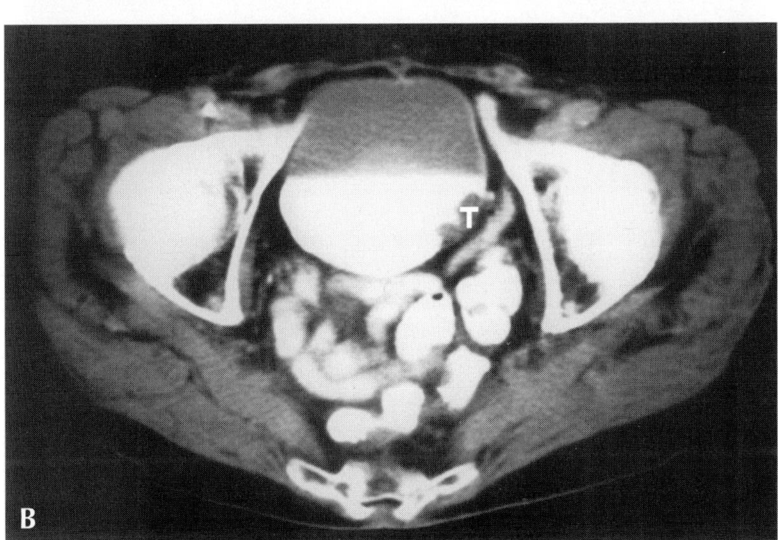

Figure 8–9. A. An intravenous urogram. A large prostate (P) indents the bladder base. A tumor (T) is present at the bladder base on the left. Bowel gas (G) projects over the bladder and should not be mistaken for a tumor. **B.** CT of the same patient shows that a tumor (T) is present along the left wall of the bladder.

dant pelvic fat will be seen. Differential diagnosis for a bladder of this shape includes large psoas muscles compressing the bladder (commonly seen in young black males), pelvic lymphadenopathy compressing the bladder, and pelvic hematomas.

ENDOMETRIOSIS

Patients with bladder endometriosis present with frequency, dysuria, hematuria, and suprapubic pain, which are cyclic with menses. At cystography a smooth elliptical defect will be seen in the bladder. Ultrasound and CT may demonstrate the mass also. Endometriosis may also affect the upper tracts, producing evidence of ureteral obstruction by IVP or ultrasound.

NEPHROGENIC ADENOMA

Chronic infection may lead to urothelial proliferation to a tissue that is similar to the proximal tubules of the nephron. This can lead to irregular bladder wall projection on cystogram or IVP. Biopsy is necessary because of radiographic similarities to carcinoma. This is not a premalignant lesion.

INFLAMMATORY BLADDER LESIONS

Cystitis may give the bladder an irregular wall. Therefore, ultrasound, cystography, or CT may demonstrate a thick-walled bladder with an irregular, ragged appearance (Fig. 8–10).

Emphysematous Cystitis

Emphysematous cystitis is a condition in which gas is present within the wall of the bladder and/or the lumen of the bladder. This usually indicates diabetes mellitus. The gas is a result of infection by *Escherichia coli* with resultant fermentation of urine glucose. This condition does not have the morbidity associated with emphysematous pyelonephritis. Radiographically, the gas causes streaky densities outlining the wall of the bladder on a plain film (Fig. 8–11). Gas may sometimes reflux up the ureters. This does not necessarily mean that the patient is prone to vesicoureteral reflux. Gas within the bladder may cause an air–fluid level when the films are obtained in the upright position. When gas is identified within the bladder but not in the bladder

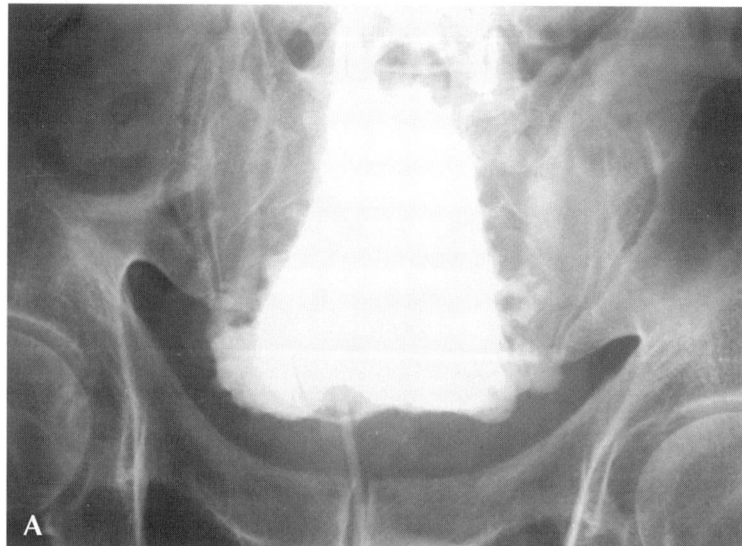

Figure 8–10. A. An intravenous urogram showing an irregular wall due to cystitis in a neurogenic bladder. **B.** A transverse ultrasound image of the bladder. The bladder wall (W) is thick and irregular.

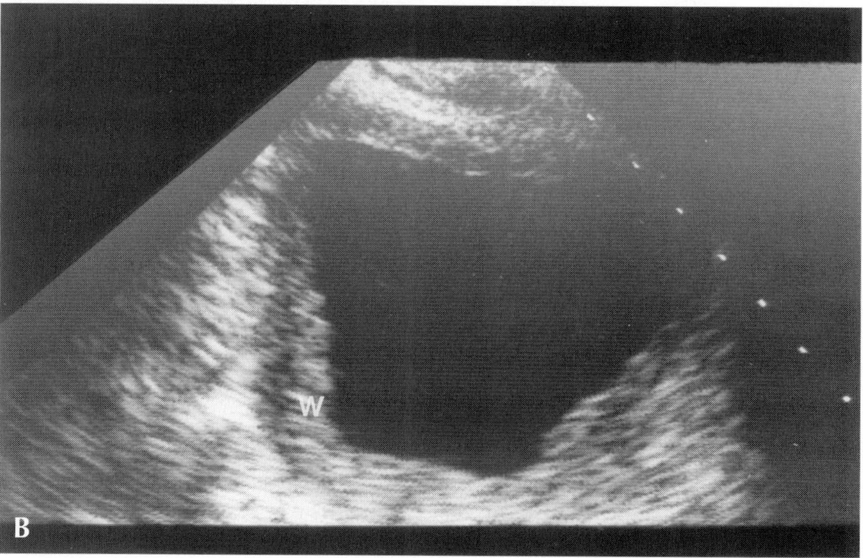

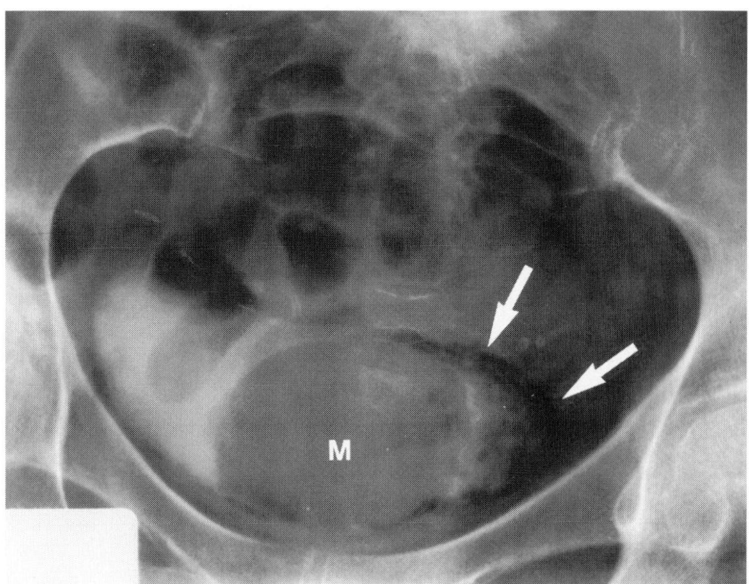

Figure 8–11. Late film from an intravenous urogram. The left bladder wall contains streaky gas (arrows). A large mass (M) is within the bladder.

wall, the possibility of fistulae between either bladder and vagina or bladder and bowel should be considered. Another cause of gas in the bladder is instrumentation with entry of gas via the urethra. Plain films show gas within the bladder and linear streaky lucencies in the wall. CT is much more sensitive and accurate for gas bubbles.

Vesicovaginal and Vesicoenteric Fistulae

Communications between bladder and bowel are often difficult to demonstrate. In addition, slightly more than half of these patients will have symptoms of pneumaturia or fecaluria. The presenting symptom may simply be polymicrobial urinary tract infection. The most common cause of this type of fistula is diverticular disease; however, colon cancer is also a frequent cause. Small-bowel fistulas to bladder may occur secondary to Crohn's disease. Trauma complications from cervical cancer and other inflammatory diseases account for the rest. Gas within the bladder is not sufficient to make a diagnosis of the presence of a fistula because the gas may occur secondary to bladder infection or secondary to recent instrumentation. Excretory urography demonstrates only a minority of these cases. Occasionally, some focal irregularity of the bladder wall will be identified. Approximately 50 percent of the cases will have contrast material that enters the bowel during cystography (Fig. 8–12). CT is much more useful for the demonstration of bladder gas and also for the demonstration of the actual fistula. CT is quite accurate at demonstrating focal bladder wall thickening.

Vesicovaginal fistulae usually present with continual dribbling of urine from the vagina. These are more often the result of radical gynecologic surgery with or without radiation therapy. Occasionally, direct invasion of the bladder by the gynecologic malignancy can be the cause of this type of fistula. Cystography is more useful in this type of fistula because the cystography may lead to opacification in the vagina. CT may also be helpful in this regard. We have on occasion pursued this diagnosis via vaginogram.

Both vesicoenteric and vesicovaginal fistulas may sometimes be diagnosed by performing a barium study of the bowel or a vaginogram with barium. Following the procedure a small sample of urine is collected. This urine is centrifuged and taken to radiology, and a radiograph of the test tube is performed. The identification of dense barium on the radiograph of the centrifuged urine confirms the presence of a fistula. This technique will not help demonstrate the location of the fistula.

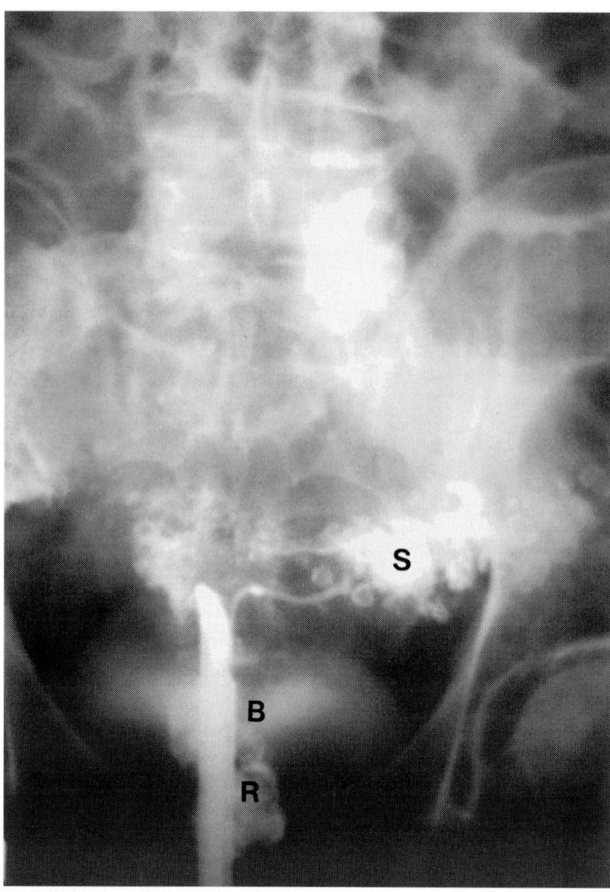

Figure 8–12. A vesicoenteric fistulogram. A cystogram showing contrast material in the bladder (B) but also contrast material in the sigmoid colon (S) and rectum (R).

Schistosomiasis

Only *S. haematobium* affects the urinary tract. This parasite is endemic in many countries, but most cases originate in North Africa or Arabia. It has an intermediate host of freshwater snails. The organism lives within the liver and portal system and excretes eggs into feces and urine. The larvae reach the liver by penetrating the skin of humans, in whom they are carried by lymphatics to the liver. The excretion of the eggs in the urine leads to the trapping of many of the eggs in the mucosa of the bladder and ureters. A severe granulomatous reaction occurs. This results in calcification of the dead eggs. Patients typically present with hematuria. As the disease advances, calcification of the entire bladder wall may be present.

Early cases of schistosomiasis have radiographic findings similar to those of other inflammatory diseases such as tuberculosis. The bladder mucosa may be inflamed with bullous edema and give an appearance on urography or cystourography of mucosal irregularity. Ultimately, portions of the bladder wall or other urothelial structures may calcify.

Initially, only segmental areas may be calcified. These patients have an increased incidence of squamous cell carcinoma, which should be suspected when plain films of the bladder reveal that formerly calcified areas are no longer calcified. Cystoscopy is usually performed to exclude squamous cell carcinoma. In this disease bladder involvement occurs before renal involvement. The most common effect on the kidneys is that of urinary obstruction (Fig. 8–13). It is common to have severe dilatation of the distal ureter on intravenous urograms. Involvement of the urethra and prostate may lead to the formation of fistula and even cavitation. Ultrasound is particularly useful for evaluating schistosomiasis because calcifications are well seen. CT is also quite good at visualizing faint calcifications. The bladder appearance on plain films may be striking because of the calcified bladder wall.

The differential diagnosis for bladder wall calcification includes not only schistosomiasis but also TB, alkaline encrustation cysts, Cytoxan cystitis, transitional cell carcinoma, squamous cell carcinoma, urachal adenocarcinoma, bladder stones, and prostatic calcifications.

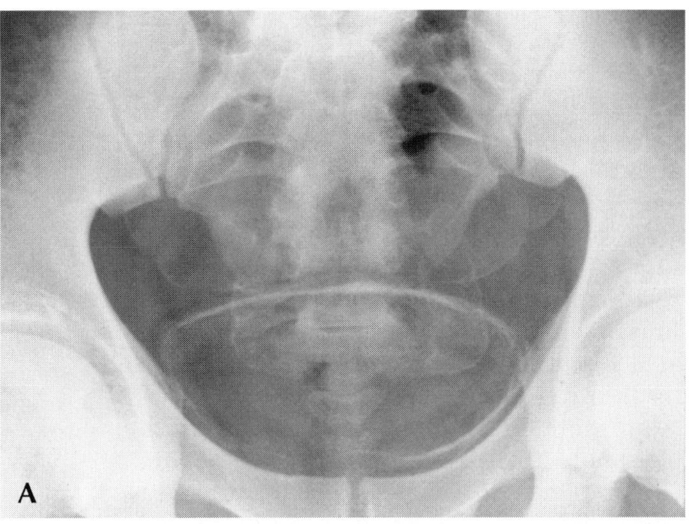

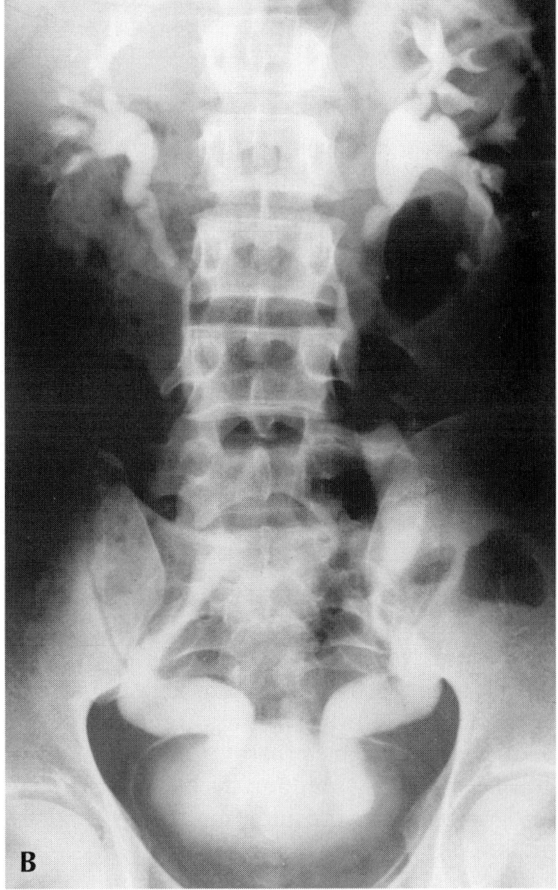

Figure 8–13. A. This plain film of the pelvis shows a calcified bladder wall due to schistosomiasis. **B.** An intravenous urogram in the same patient shows bilateral ureteric obstruction.

Bladder Stones

Bladder stones may be secondary to multiple causes, including infection, continuous or intermittent bladder catherization, schistosomiasis, bladder outlet obstruction, foreign bodies, migration from the kidneys, and endemic calculi.

About one-third of bladder stones occur as a result of bladder infection, usually from *E. coli* or *Proteus mirabilis.* Calcium oxalate is frequently associated with *E. coli.* Calcium phosphate carbonate is more often associated with *P. mirabilis.* Infections may produce stones that are composed of calcium oxalate, calcium phosphate, or varying mixtures of these. Urease-producing organisms, such as *P. mirabilis* or *Klebsiella* spp., may cause stones that contain a matrix material as a result of debris coming from the urethral lining of the ureter or bladder. Magnesium ammonium phosphate and calcium phosphate carbonate (struvite and carbonate apatite) are sometimes referred to as urea stones. These stones are poorly mineralized because of the presence of the matrix and therefore are poorly seen radiographically.

Stones may also be associated with bladder catheters. Indwelling catheters will ultimately lead to bacterial infections and may cause magnesium ammonium phosphate stones as well as calcium oxalate and phosphate stones. Debris forms on the balloon of the catheter, and this debris may act as a nidus for stone formation. This is particularly true in neurogenic bladders. In addition, intermittent catheterization may introduce pubic hairs and other foreign bodies even if good technique is followed. These pubic hairs may act as a nidus for stones in the bladder.

In schistosomiasis stones may form in the bladder as a result of bladder neck obstruction. The stones are not the direct result of the calcification in the wall or of the parasitic worm. The bladder neck obstruction occurs because of fibrosis.

About two-thirds of bladder stones in adults are a result of bladder outlet obstruction. This usually occurs secondary to enlargement of the prostate gland, but urethral strictures, bladder neck hypertrophy, and neurogenic bladder may also lead to outlet obstruction. These stones may be composed of calcium oxalate, calcium phosphate, uric acid, cystine, or calcium carbonate. Foreign bodies may lead to a nidus for stone formation. Migrating sutures that have been placed in the bladder wall are an example of such a nidus. Patients who introduce foreign bodies to their urethra may also present with stones.

Idiopathic endemic calculi occur in young children in third-world countries. These stones were formerly seen in Europe and the United States prior to World War II. Such stones may be a result of low levels of phosphate in the diet and may occur when milk is discontinued early in infancy.

Radiographically, pure uric acid stones will not be visualized on a plain film. Magnesium ammonium phosphate and calcium phosphate carbonate are faintly radiopaque. In general, the stones that contain calcium are better seen than stones that do not have calcium (Fig. 8–14). Contrast material in the bladder may obscure a stone at excretory urography. However, careful examination of images of the bladder may show a negative filling defect (Fig. 8–15). Ultrasound and CT will detect the stones regardless of their composition. Even the radiolucent uric acid stones will present as high-density areas on a CT scan. These stones should cast a shadow at ultrasound (Fig. 8–16), and at ultrasound the presence of the shadow is one way to distinguish a bladder stone from a soft tissue bladder mass.

Tuberculosis of the Bladder

Genitourinary tuberculosis affects the kidneys but may affect the bladder as well. The bladder mucosa shows bullous changes and becomes contracted and irregular. Calcification may occur late in the process. The bladder becomes stiff, which may cause incompetent intramural tunnels, ureterovesical junction obstruction, and secondary reflux.

ALKALINE ENCRUSTATION CYSTITIS

Sheets of calcium occur on damaged bladder urothelium. For this to occur, the urine must be alkaline and chronic infection with *P. mirabilis* is usually a precursor.

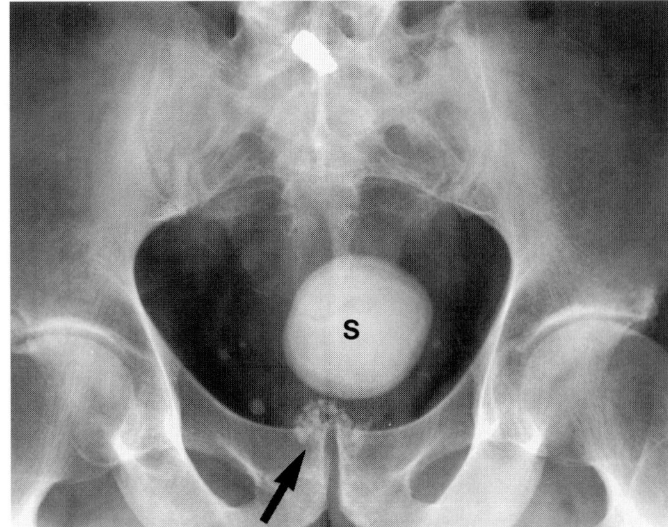

Figure 8–14. A patient with a large calcified bladder stone (S). Prostate calcifications are also noted (arrow).

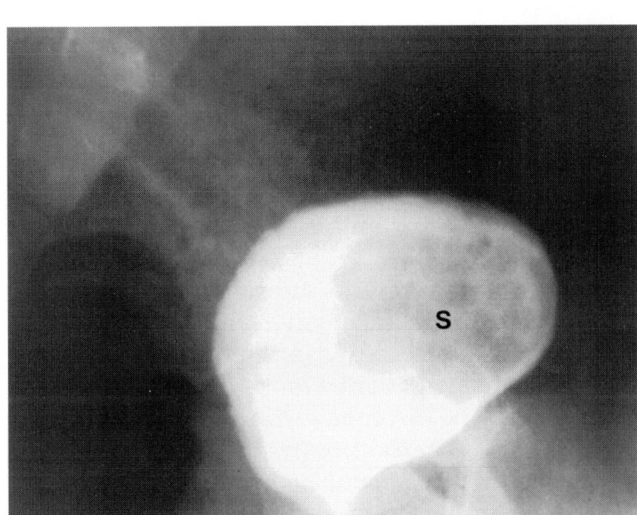

Figure 8–15. A cystogram. This lateral film shows a negative defect due to a large stone (S).

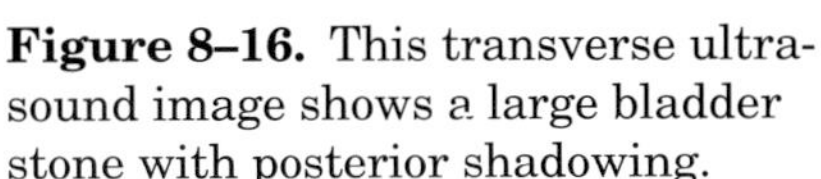

Figure 8–16. This transverse ultrasound image shows a large bladder stone with posterior shadowing.

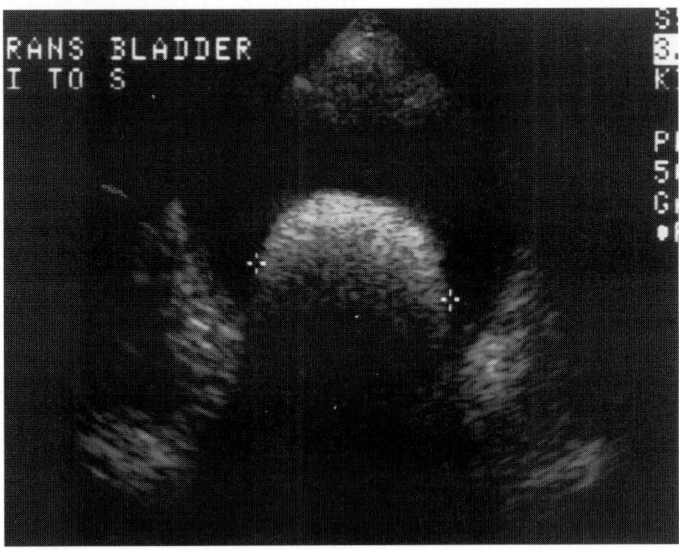

CYSTITIS CYSTICA

This entity occurs in females who have chronic or recurrent bladder infection. Rests of transitional epithelium degenerate, and blebs form in the bladder wall. These blebs are serous cysts. They are usually only millimeters in diameter but may reach a size of 1 to 2 cm. They are more numerous at the bladder base. Radiographically, they produce multiple smooth filling defects. They are not premalignant.

CYSTITIS GLANDULARIS

Hypertrophy of mucous-secreting glands occurs, probably as a result of chronic infection. Multiple irregular filling defects are seen. The differential diagnosis includes transitional cell carcinoma. This lesion is premalignant.

SQUAMOUS METAPLASIA

Another response to chronic irritation or infection is metaplasia of urothelium to a squamous type. Leukoplakia may form. Rarely, a malignant degeneration to squamous cell carcinoma may occur. Radiographically, wall irregularity, filling defects, or masses may be seen.

MALACOPLAKIA

This is a lesion usually seen in females and also is associated with chronic infection or irritation. The lesions occur due to the inability of macrophages to effectively digest bacteria, causing the formation of intracellular inclusions known as Michaelis-Guttman bodies. This leads to plaque formation. Radiographically, multiple filling defects usually are seen in the bladder base. These filling defects are smooth.

BLADDER RUPTURE

Bladder rupture can be caused by penetrating, blunt, or iatrogenic trauma. Over 80 percent of bladder ruptures have associated pelvic fractures. However, when pelvic fractures are seen, only about 10 percent of the time is there an associated bladder rupture. The full bladder is more vulnerable to rupture than an empty bladder. Rupture at the dome, the weakest part of the bladder, results in intraperitoneal extravasation of urine (Fig. 8–17). This type of injury requires surgical intervention. Extraperitoneal rupture is frequently associated with fractures of the pubic rami (Fig. 8–18). More than 80 percent of the time when there is a pelvic fracture with coexistent bladder rupture, the bladder rupture will be extraperitoneal. In this situation, the tear is close to the neck of the bladder. In approximately 10 percent of cases, there may be combined intra- and extraperitoneal rupture of the bladder. Symptoms of bladder rupture include suprapubic gross tenderness and hematuria.

Cystography is the radiographic test of choice, with a sensitivity of 85 to 100 percent. Negative cystograms may occur because the rent has sealed. The bladder should be distended with a minimum of 300 mL of 30 percent contrast. If there is a Foley catheter, it should be clamped. It is important to do a radiograph of the bladder after the contrast is drained. Ten percent of ruptures will be diagnosed on this film only (Fig. 8–19). Computed tomography of the bladder is not adequate unless the CT is done similar to cystography with adequate distention of the bladder and clamping of the Foley catheter. An intravenous urogram is not a substitute for cystography. Associated pelvic hematomas may give a pear-shaped appearance to the bladder due to lateral compression from the hematoma. If the base of the bladder is elevated above the symphysis, a urethral injury should be suspected. The radiographic appearance of an intraperitoneal rupture consists of contrast in the peritoneal cavity, which outlines bowel loops and extends up the paracolic gutters to the visceral organs. It may be helpful to put the patient in a Trendelenburg position to facili-

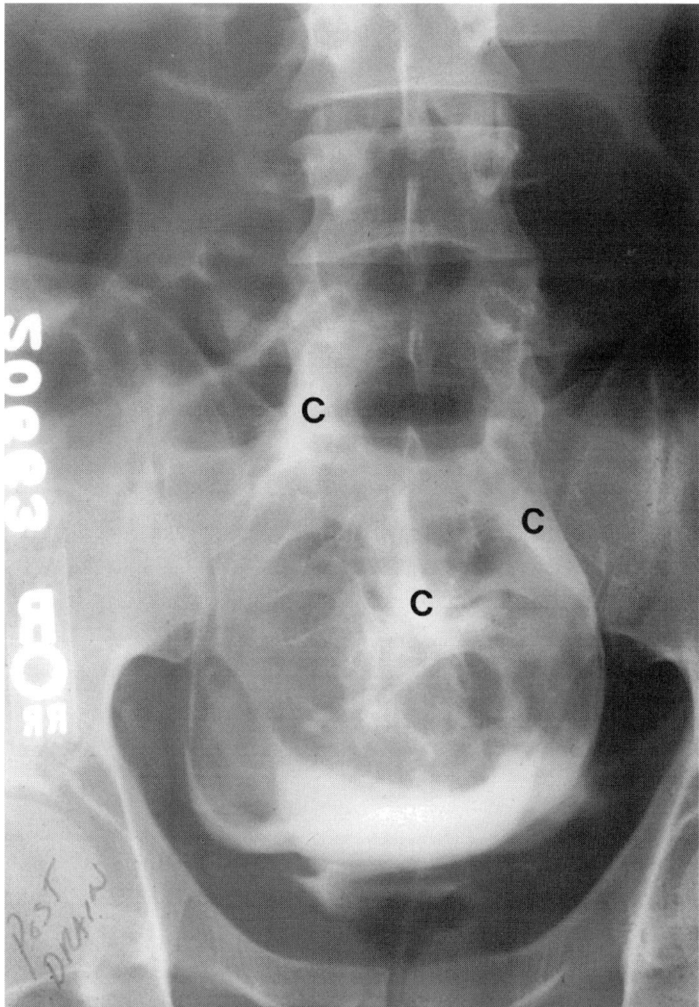

Figure 8–17. This postcystogram film shows contrast material (C) extending into the intraperitoneal spaces and the surrounding bowel.

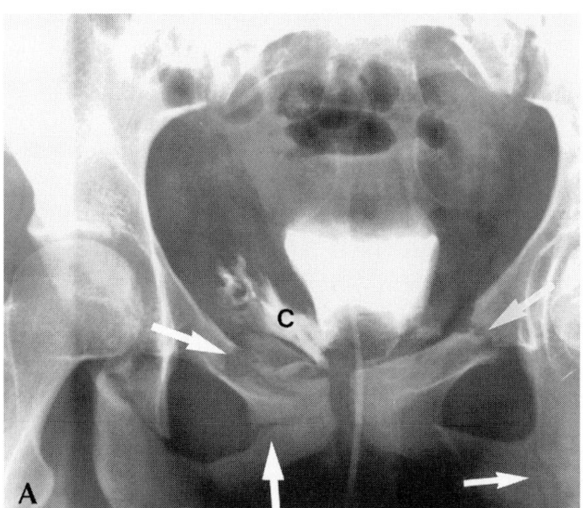

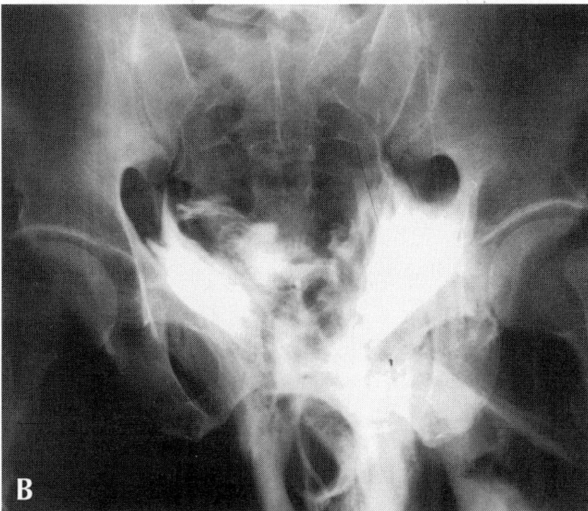

Figure 8–18. A. This cystogram shows an extraperitoneal bladder rupture (C) in this patient with pelvic fractures (arrows). The contrast material streaks in the extraperitoneal spaces around the bladder. **B.** Postdrainage film shows a large amount of leaked contrast. Contrast is leaking into the perineum, suggesting disruption of the genitourinary diaphragm and/or urethra.

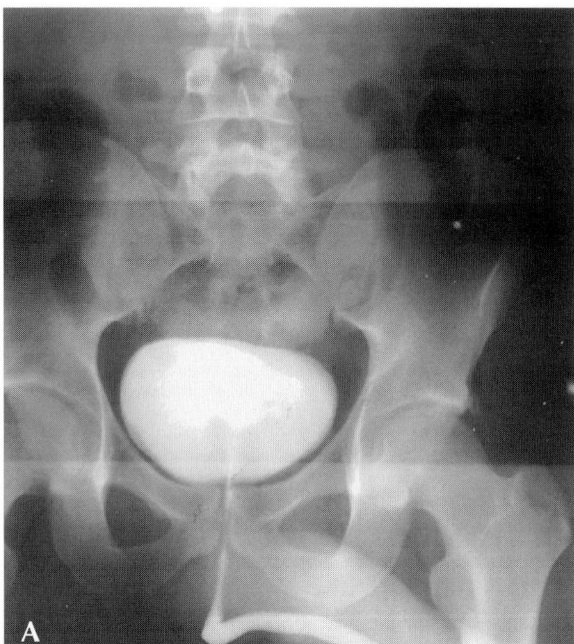

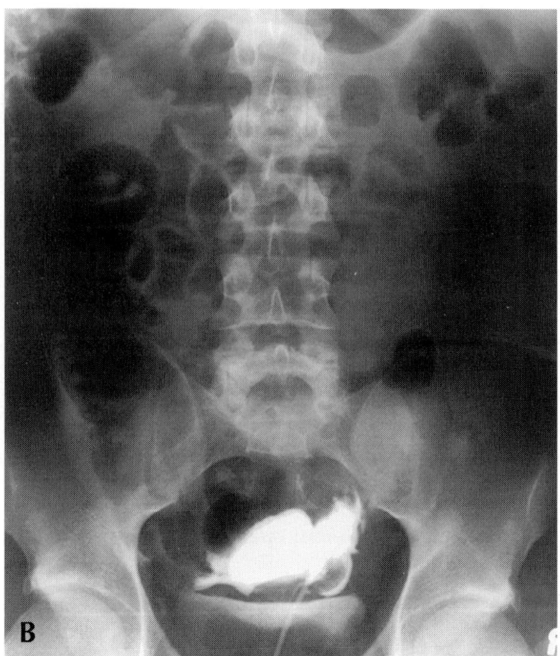

Figure 8–19. A. A cystogram in another patient. The bladder appears intact. **B.** This postdrainage film shows extravesicular contrast material, indicating bladder rupture.

tate movement of contrast up the gutters and around the spleen or other viscera.

For extraperitoneal rupture, streaky or "flame" patterns of contrast material will be seen on a cystogram with the contrast material tracking laterally and superiorly in the preperitoneal and retroperitoneal space (Figs. 8–18, 8–19). This injury can usually be managed conservatively with placement of a Foley catheter. If the GU diaphragm is disrupted, there may be contrast material extending into the thigh, scrotum, and perineum (Fig. 8–18*B*). If a urethral disruption has necessitated placement of a suprapubic catheter, it is important to do a cystogram to rule out an associated rupture of the bladder.

Chapter

9

Prostate

NORMAL PROSTATE ULTRASOUND

Prostate ultrasound is performed with either a 5- or 7-MHz endorectal transducer. A condom is placed over the transducer. Either a water bath or lubricating gel is placed between the transducer and the condom to maintain good contact with the transducer. This provides acoustic coupling.

The prostate gland is divided histologically into four zones (Fig. 9–1). The transitional zone is adjacent to the urethra and is the site of benign prostatic hypertrophy. The peripheral zone accounts for the largest portion of the prostate gland and lies peripherally and next to the rectum. Approximately 70 percent of prostate cancers originate from this area. The central zone is located at the superior portion of the prostate. A fibromuscular zone known as the anterior stroma lies anterior to the urethra.

Visualization of the zonal anatomy requires state-of-the-art, high-resolution ultrasound equipment. No cleansing enema is required. If biopsy is planned, coverage with antibiotics must occur. Three doses of ciproflaxacin commencing the night before the biopsy is one regimen. There is a risk of sepsis and even death if coverage is inadequate. The gland is scanned in the sagittal and longitudinal planes. Any asymmetry of the seminal vesicles is noted. Obliteration or invasion of the fat between the prostate and the seminal vesicles suggests invasion by tumor. The peripheral borders of the prostate are examined for evidence that tumor is invading outward from the prostate into the periprostatic fat.

The cephalad portion of the prostate abutting the bladder neck is also known as the base. The ejaculatory ducts pass through this region and connect the seminal vesicle to the urethra. The seminal vesicles may be identified at the base of the prostate gland (Fig. 9–2). In the axial plane they resemble a bow tie, and in the sagittal plane they resemble a projection sticking off the base of the prostate. The apex of the prostate gland is located inferiorly. Multiple images should be obtained in both the sagittal and transverse planes. The overall size and shape of the glands should be evaluated.

Hypoechoic areas in the prostate can be indicative of prostate cancer. Significant numbers of prostate cancers may be hyper- or isoechoic. Therefore, there is controversy as to whether biopsies of hypoechoic areas are more useful than random biopsies. The seminal vesicles should be symmetric in shape.

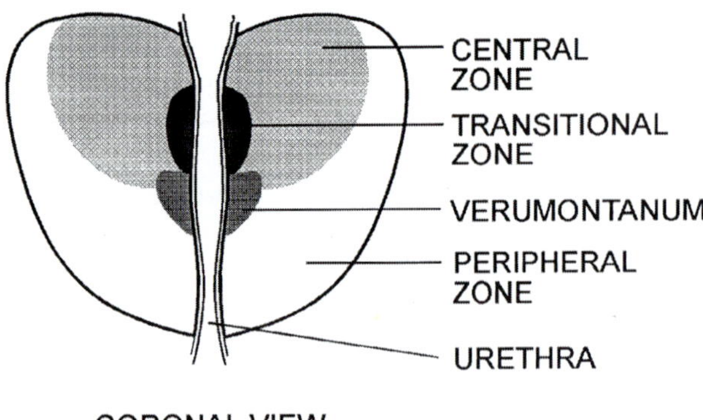

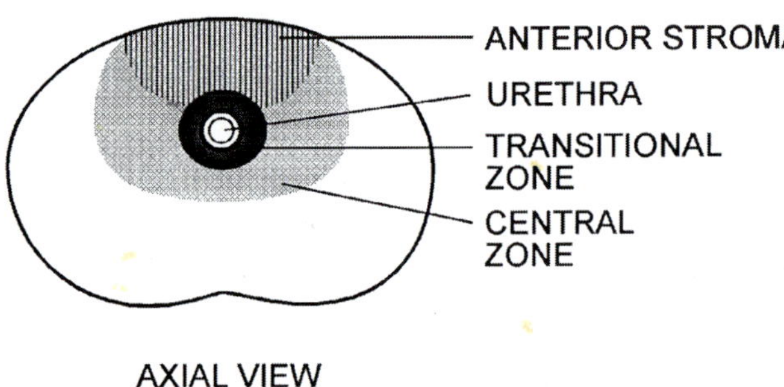

Figure 9–1. A schematic drawing of the zonal anatomy of the prostate in the coronal and axial planes. The nonshaded area is the peripheral zone.

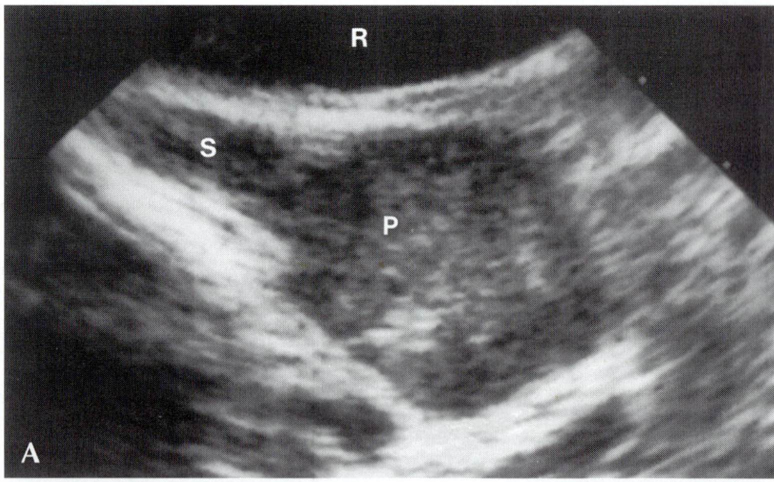

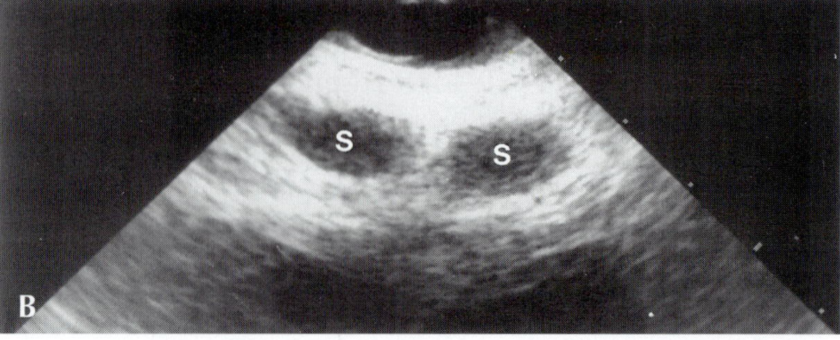

Figure 9–2. A. A sagittal image of the prostate showing the prostate (P) and the seminal vesicles (S). R = rectum. **B.** Transverse images of the seminal vesicles (S).

Calcifications appear in the glands as hyperechoic areas with acoustic shadows behind them. Corpora amylacea present as hyperechoic areas in the prostate without shadowing. Corpora amylacea are the result of inspissated secretions formed from glycoproteins. It is common to see cysts in the prostate. There are some congenital cysts (including utricle cysts) in the region of the verumontanum, Müllerian duct cysts that are near the midline, and ejaculatory duct cysts that are a result of dilatation of the ejaculatory duct. Cysts in the parenchyma of the prostate may be postinflammatory and are the most common cysts imaged.

MAGNETIC RESONANCE IMAGING OF THE PROSTATE

Magnetic resonance imaging of the prostate, so far, has been disappointing. Attempts have been made to use MRI for screening in an effort to see if MRI can detect cancers. Attempts have also been made to use MRI for staging prostate carcinoma using endorectal coils.

Normal MRI shows a homogeneous-appearing gland on T1-weighted images. The fat around the prostate is relatively high in signal compared to the prostate gland itself. Tortuous structures may represent vessels in the periprostatic fat. Seminal vesicles are of low signal intensity on T1-weighted images. On T2-weighted images, the central zone is of lower intensity than the surrounding peripheral zone. The anterior fibromuscular zone is also of low signal intensity. The prostatic urethra and periurethral glands may appear high in signal intensity compared to the surrounding central zone.

A thin, low-signal area, which is thought to represent the prostatic capsule, will appear on both T1- and T2-weighted images. Seminal vesicles will have high signal intensity on a T2-weighted image. Because of the appearance of the different parts of the prostate on T2-weighted imaging, this technique is most useful for delineating abnormalities. Benign prostatic hypertrophy (BPH) may appear heterogeneous or may have a homogeneous appearance on T1-weighted images. T2-weighted images may show enlargement of the inner portion of the prostate in BPH with discrete nodules of either high or low signal intensity. Areas of high signal intensity may be scattered throughout the gland secondary to either hemorrhage or cyst formation.

Prostate cancer usually appears as an area of low signal intensity on T2-weighted images (Fig. 9–3) when compared to the adjacent peripheral zone. In the central zone prostate cancer is difficult to detect. The lesion will usually not be seen on a T1-weighted image. Prostate cancers cannot be distinguished from BPH. Only 60 percent of lesions larger than 5 mm will be identified on MRI. In addition, there may be other causes of low-signal intensity areas in the peripheral zone, such as chronic prostatitis or atrophy. MRI imaging is not a sensitive method for detecting prostate cancer. The accuracy of MRI for staging prostate cancer has been shown to be about 60 percent, similar to CT. Therefore, the exact role of MRI

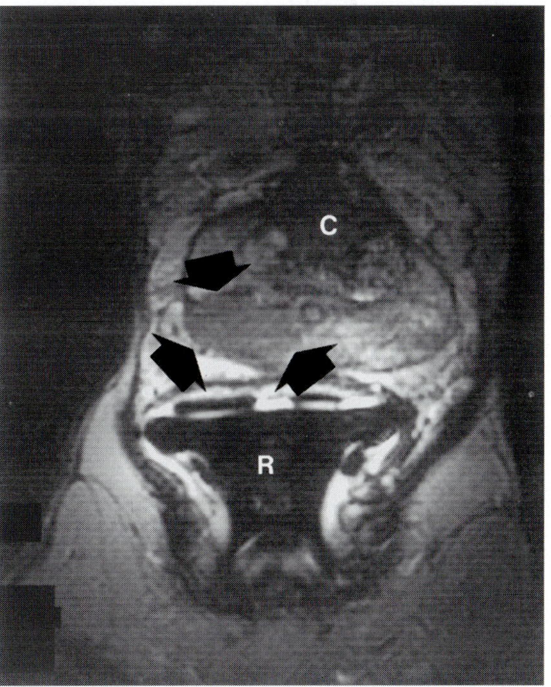

Figure 9–3. MRI of the prostate Central zone = C. Arrows demarcate abnormal signal of cancer. R = rectum. (Courtesy of Dr. Paul Ross, University of Colorado Health Sciences Center, Denver, CO)

in evaluating the prostate gland is unclear at this time.

PROSTATIC CALCULI

Calcification of the prostate may occur in areas of the corpora amylacea (Fig. 9–4). These calcifications may be seen on plain films. Calcification also occurs in patients with carcinomas, with adenomas, and with necrotic areas for other reasons, such as infection. In particular, tuberculosis and schistosomiasis of the prostate may lead to extensive calcifications. Only about 5 percent of prostate carcinomas will calcify.

Another situation in which prostatic calcification occurs is in patients with hyperreflexive neurogenic bladder. This abnormality occurs when the neural lesion is above the level of the sacrum and the brain stem micturition center is disconnected from the sacral cord. These patients have a spastic bladder. The common causes are multiple sclerosis, myelodysplasia, spinal cord trauma, spinal cord tumors, and herniated intervertebral disks. At voiding, these patients have no coordination between the bladder and the urethral sphincter, causing high bladder pressure. High pressures may lead to reflux of urine into prostatic ducts and can ultimately lead to multiple prostatic calculi.

BENIGN PROSTATIC HYPERTROPHY ON ULTRASOUND

Benign prostatic hypertrophy (BPH) usually develops from the transitional zone of the prostate, although occasionally it develops from the periurethral glands. With imaging, the urethra may be compressed laterally and deviated posteriorly. At transrectal sonography adenomas may be seen to cause a bulge of the contour of the prostate. The prostate becomes more oval or round. Occasionally, there may be asymmetrical enlargement of the prostate. Echotexture of the prostate may be heterogeneous or homogeneous. Small calculi may be identified. Since the ultrasonographic central zone is the portion of the prostate that is enlarged, sagittal scans are better for visualizing BPH. It may not be possible with ultrasound to distinguish between the internal

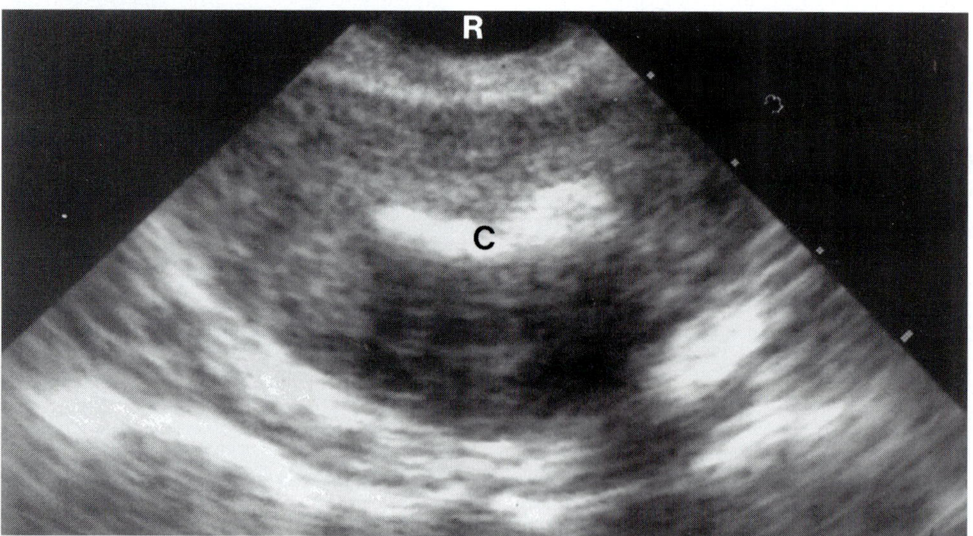

Figure 9–4. This tranverse ultrasound image of the prostate shows a large calcification (C). R = rectum.

portions of the gland, where BPH occurs, and the external, more peripheral, portions of the prostate, which are at greater risk for developing cancer.

PROSTATE CANCER

At transrectal sonography, the classic appearance of prostate cancer is that of a hypoechoic area in the peripheral zone (Fig. 9–5). However, only 70 percent of prostate carcinomas occur in the peripheral zone. Not all prostate carcinomas are hypoechoic. Significant numbers of cancers will be isoechoic or hyperechoic. The cause of the variable appearance is unclear. In a histologic study of prostate specimens, the ultrasound appearance of prostate cancer was hypoechoic or slightly hyperechoic in 30 to 76 percent of cancers. The lesion was isoechoic in 24 to 57 percent and hypoechoic or mixed in about 15 percent.

There has been an attempt to correlate the ultrasound appearance with the grade of the tumor. Well-differentiated carcinomas and intermediate-grade tumors have a greater tendency to be hypoechoic. When prostate ultrasound is performed, areas of asymmetry or unusual echotexture should be biopsied.

Staging of prostate carcinoma by CT has been studied, with reported accuracies of 67 to 77 percent, sensitivities of 33 to 50 percent, and specificities of 75 to 100 percent. Prostate cancer is staged by the schema in Table 9–1. However, CT cannot differentiate Stage A (T1) from Stage B (T2). In separating Stage B from Stage C, CT has an accuracy of about 60 percent. Computed tomography is most useful in detecting gross metastatic disease and separating Stage D from Stage C disease (Fig. 9–6) and should be used when there is high probability of advanced disease.

Magnetic resonance imaging has been attempted for staging prostate carcinoma, but these results have been disappointing and similar to or slightly better than CT. This is true even when endorectal coils are used.

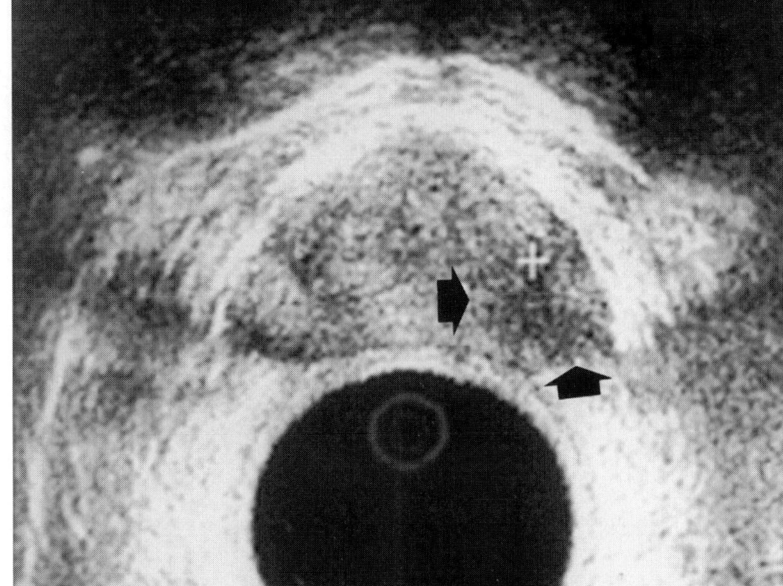

Figure 9–5. This transverse ultrasound image of the prostate shows hypoechoic prostate cancer (arrows).

TABLE 9–1. **American Urological Association Staging System for Prostate Cancer**

Stage		Characteristics
A		Occult cancer
	A1	Focal diffuse
	A2	Diffuse
B		Cancer confined within the prostatic capsule with no elevation of serum acid phosphatase
	B1	Tumor <1.5 or 1 lobe
	B2	Tumor >1.5 cm or >1 lobe
C		Cancer extending beyond the prostatic capsule, including seminal vesicles, bladder, and urethra, or confined within the capsule with elevated serum acid phosphatase
	C1	No involvement of seminal vesicles
	C2	Involvement of seminal vesicles
D		Metastatic disease
	D1	Pelvic lymph node metastases
	D2	Bone or distant lymph node or organ metastases

Data from Whitmore WF Jr: Natural History and Staging of Prostate Cancer. *Urol Clin North Am* 11:205, 1984.

Prostate Cancer Bone Metastases and Cord Compression

Spinal cord compression may occur as a result of metastatic disease to the spine. The sacrum is more often involved than the thoracic or lumbar spine. Metastases are more often osteolytic, such as occur with lung, breast, and kidney primaries. On plain film, prostate cancers usually have osteosclerotic metastatic disease (Fig. 9–7). This is different from other cancers, such as lung or kidney cancer, which cause mostly osteolytic metastases. Plain films will pick up approximately one-third of metastases to the spine. One of the classic radiographic presentations of metastatic prostate disease is an ivory vertebral body—a single vertebral body that is extremely dense on a plain radiograph. Magnetic resonance imaging is particularly good at showing the extent of narrowing of the spinal canal and compression of the cord. Computed tomography is better at showing bony involvement of the spinal canal. Computed tomographic myel-

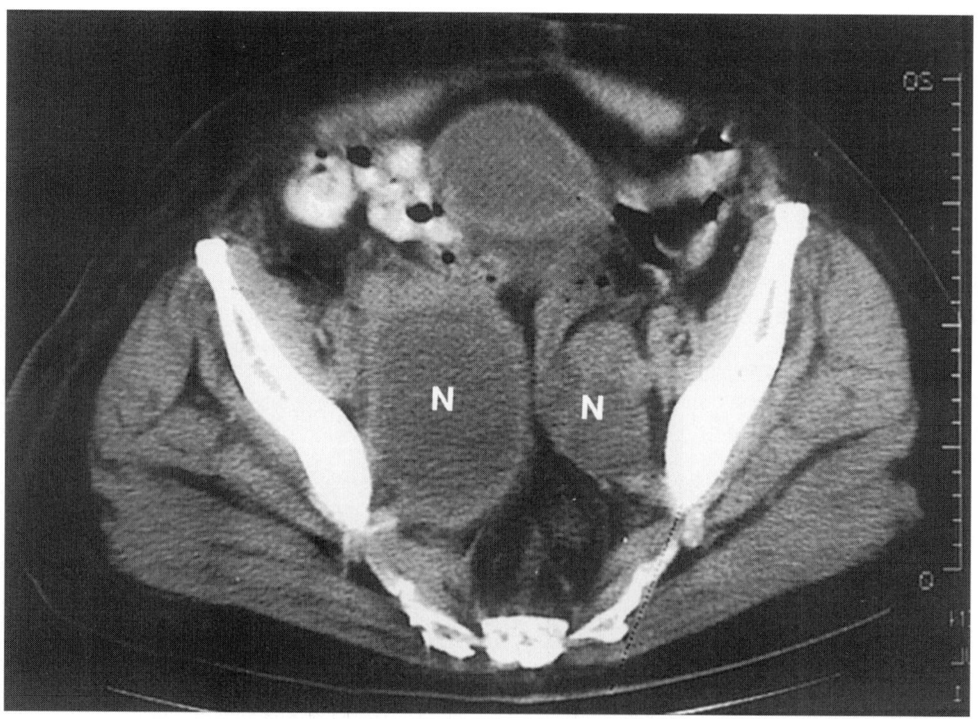

Figure 9–6. CT of the pelvis showing stage D1 disease. Large necrotic nodes = N.

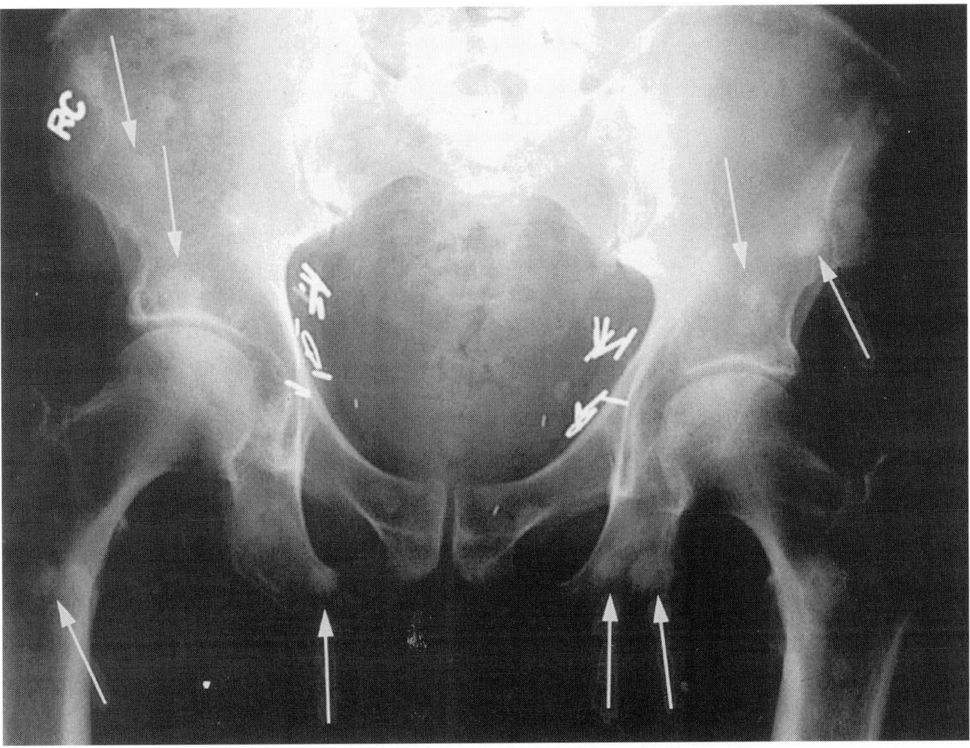

Figure 9–7. Plain film of the pelvis showing sclerotic metastases (arrows) to bone.

ography may occasionally be useful, but it has largely been replaced by MRI.

Prostate cancer most often metastasizes to the lumbosacral spine and bony pelvis tissue before spreading to more distal bones. Bone scanning is the test of choice (Fig. 9–8). Because of similarities to Paget's disease of the bone, it is important to be aware of the characteristics of this relatively benign disease.

Paget's Disease

Paget's disease may need to be excluded as a cause of abnormalities or bone scan or plain film in a patient with prostate cancer. The cause of Paget's disease is unknown and is characterized by excessive and aggressive remodeling of bone with very active bone resorption and formation. Therefore, Paget's disease is a combination of osteoclastic and osteoblastic activity. The radiographic appearance is secondary to the osseous resorption and laying down of new bone. In Paget's disease, there is an increase in blood flow to the bone with increased proximate skin temperature.

The disease can go through multiple stages of osteoclastic and osteoblastic activity. The vertebral column is commonly involved, which may cause collapse of vertebral bodies. The mass of Pagetic bone may interfere with the blood supply to the spinal cord. In addition, the new bone may result in stenosis of neuroforamina. On plain film, the trabeculae of the bone in Paget's disease become enlarged and prominent. The appearance of the vertebral body in Paget's disease may resemble a "picture frame." The periphery of the vertebral body will have a very thick and dense appearance. Sometimes Paget's disease may cause an ivory vertebral body similar to that seen in metastatic disease from prostate carcinoma. In the pelvis there may be trabecular thickening with sclerosis around the inner margins of the pelvis. Sclerosis may be adjacent to the sacroiliac joint and also around the

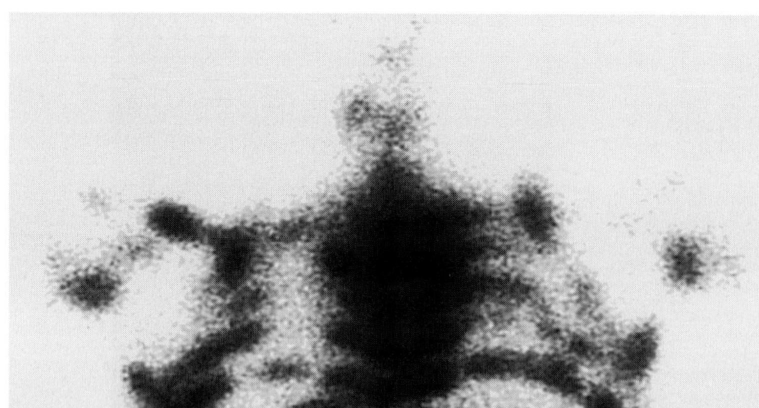

Figure 9–8. Posterior bone scan image of the thorax showing widespread metastatic disease.

periphery of the iliac bone. There is a tendency to involve the epiphysis of the long bone. The bone may be enlarged and deformed with the coarse trabeculae. The cortical bone may be thickened. There may be radiolucent areas of varying size intermixed with the coarse sclerotic bone. On a bone scan, Paget's disease will be extremely hot (Fig. 9–9). Paget's disease has a typical distribution that is asymmetric or unilateral, which is more typical of Paget's disease than osteoblastic metastatic disease. Ultimately, the distinction between prostate metastases and Paget's disease may require a plain x ray of the pelvis.

PROSTATE ABSCESS

Prostate abscess is usually a result of progression of prostatitis and formation of a frank abscess cavity. It usually occurs in men in their 40s and 50s who present with high fevers and pain in the region of the perineum. They may have difficulty voiding. Diabetics are predisposed to this problem. Prostatic abscess is usually diagnosed clinically, aided by digital rectal examination. At CT there is usually a single irregular low-density area within the prostate. Computed tomography is most useful in defining the extent of the abscess. Transrectal sonography may show a hypoechoic irregular area within the prostate, usually containing debris.

DILATED PROSTATIC UTRICLE

The prostatic utricle is a remnant of the Müllerian duct. The other vestigial remnant of the Müllerian duct is the appendix of the testes. The Müllerian duct does not atrophy. The result may be formation of cysts along the route of the vas deferens from the scrotum to the ejaculatory ducts. The utricle is a Müllerian remnant that usually occurs as a small cystic cavity in the central verumontanum. Dilated utricles can be seen from infancy into adolescence. They are often

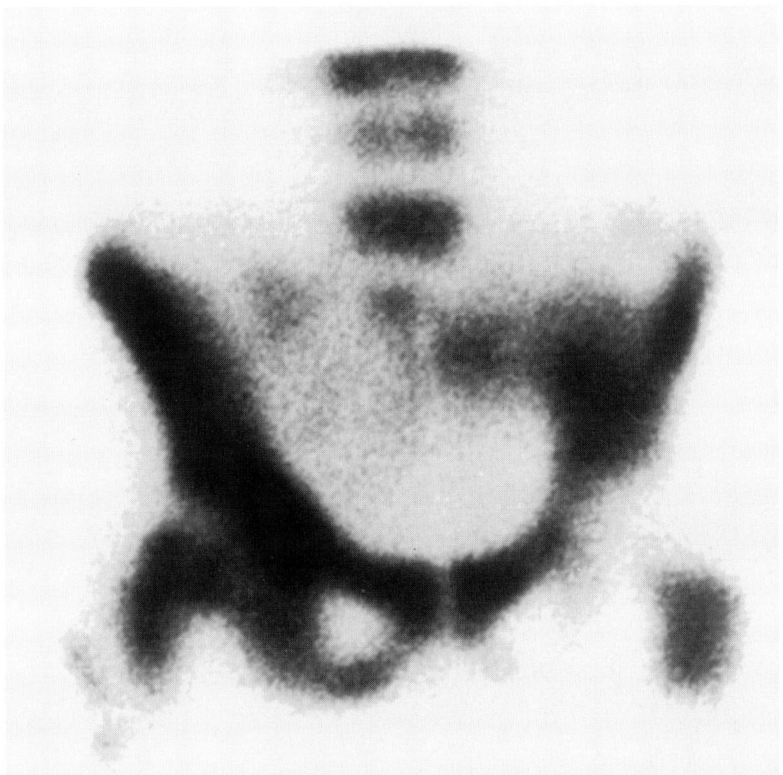

Figure 9–9. A bone scan of the pelvis in Paget's disease.

associated with hypospadias and cryptorchidism. Radiographically, they are seen on voiding cystourethrograms. They will be filled in a retrograde fashion, and the films will show the cavity containing the contrast material that extends from the verumontanum posteriorly into the prostatic urethra. These are seen in a few percent of patients during prostate ultrasound.

SEMINAL VESICLE CYSTS

Cysts of the seminal vesicle may be appreciated during prostate ultrasound or may be seen during pelvic ultrasound, CT, or MRI of the pelvis. Embryologically, the ureteral bud and seminal vesicle derive from the mesonephric duct. If the ureteral bud does not develop properly, renal agenesis may result. Renal agenesis plus genital abnormalities (such as seminal vesicle cysts) may occur if the mesonephric duct fails to develop. Therefore, 60 to 70 percent of seminal vesicle cysts have associated renal agenesis. Confusion may arise from ectopic ureteral insertion into the seminal vesicle. Müllerian duct cysts may also cause confusion.

Absence of the seminal vesicle plus absence of the vas deferens may also be associated with renal agenesis.

Chapter

10

Urethra

NORMAL RETROGRADE URETHROGRAM

The posterior urethra starts at the bladder neck and extends to the distal urogenital diaphragm (Fig. 10–1*A*). The posterior urethra is divided into a proximal prostatic portion and a distal membranous portion. The anterior urethra consists of a proximal bulbous portion that extends from the distal urogenital diaphragm to the penoscrotal junction and a penile portion that extends from the penoscrotal junction to the external meatus. The fossa navicularis is the dilated portion of the urethra just proximal to the external meatus.

To perform a retrograde urethrogram, a Foley catheter is inserted about 2 cm into the penis. The balloon is inflated slightly with 1 to 2 mL of saline. The balloon is thereby lodged in the fossa navicularis. Contrast material (30 percent iodine) is injected as mild traction is applied. Several films are obtained during retrograde injection. The bladder is then filled, the catheter is usually removed, and the patient is instructed to void while several more films are obtained. In trauma, often only the retrograde portion of the study is obtained.

In a male the membranous urethra can be radiographically delineated as that section of urethra between the distal end of the verumontanum and the proximal end of the dilated bulbous urethra (Fig. 10–1*B*). The bulbous urethra forms a very typical-appearing cone. It is the proximal end of this cone that demarcates the beginning of the bulbous urethra and the end of the membranous urethra. The verumontanum lies in the posterior wall of the prostatic urethra. In the midline of the proximal verumontanum is the orifice of the prostatic utricle, which is a vestige of the Müllerian duct. The ejaculatory ducts open on either side of the verumontanum.

The female urethra (Fig. 10–1*B*) is quite different from the male urethra. The female urethra measures approximately 2.5 to 4 cm long, whereas the male urethra measures between 15 and 19 cm. The female urethra also shows more variability in shape and appearance.

CONGENITAL ABNORMALITIES

Urethral Duplication

Urethral duplication is divided into complete versus incomplete. In complete duplication there is an extra urethra that has its own

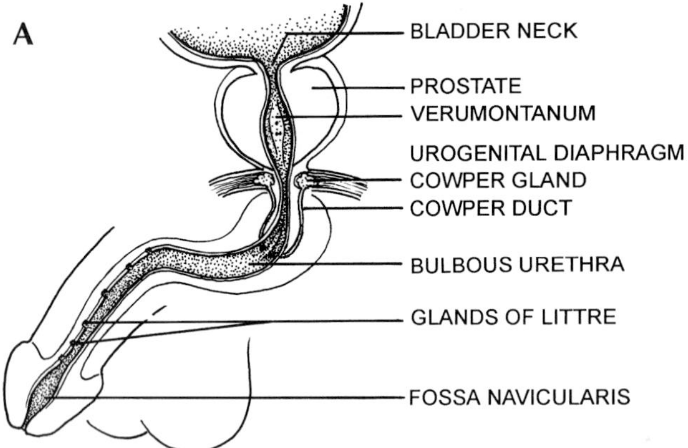

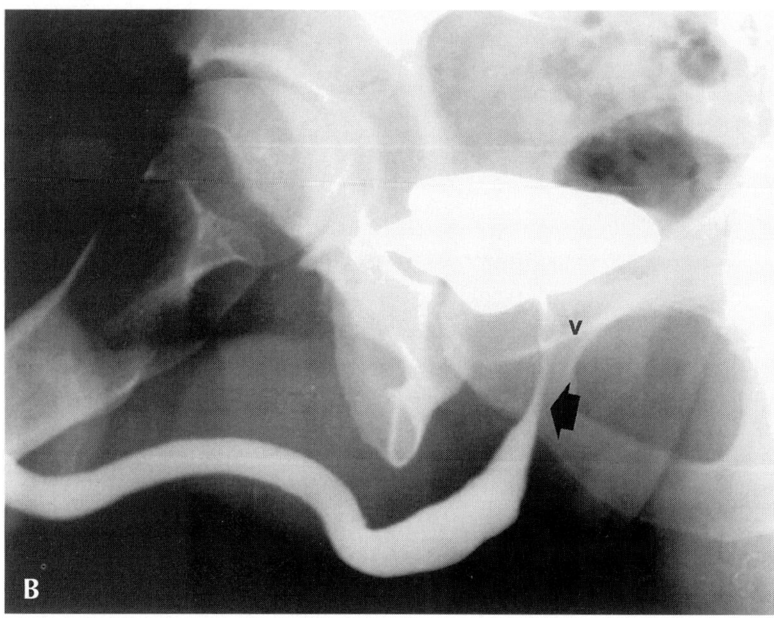

Figure 10–1. A. A diagram of a male urethra. **B.** A urethrogram. V is next to the verumontanum of the prostatic urethra. From the distal verumontanum to the beginning of the cone (arrow) is the membranous urethra. The arrow marks the beginning of the cone-shaped bulbous urethra. **C.** A diagram of a female urethra.

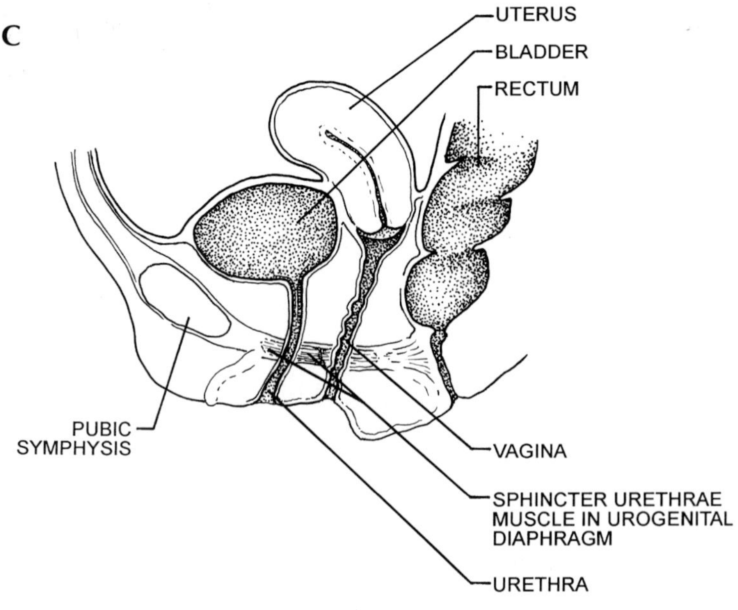

opening into the bladder and has its own meatus in the distal penis. This may be associated with either bladder duplication or penile duplication. In males the two urethras lie one above the other (Fig. 10–2*A*), although in females they may be side by side. The extra urethra may not have normal sphincter mechanisms, and therefore the patient may present with incontinence. The extra meatus may be either epispadic or hypospadic.

With incomplete duplication the double urethra may either be distal or proximal. That is, the urethra may have a takeoff point from a normal urethra (Fig. 10–2). Only one urethra will exit from the bladder. An extra meatus may occur in a hypospadic position. Patients may also have an accessory urethra. This is a type of incomplete duplication, but the accessory urethra does not communicate with either the bladder or urethra. This accessory urethra is subject to infection. Radiologically, all urethral orifices should be studied in a retrograde fashion. In rare circumstances, an accessory urethra may arise from the normal urethra and not

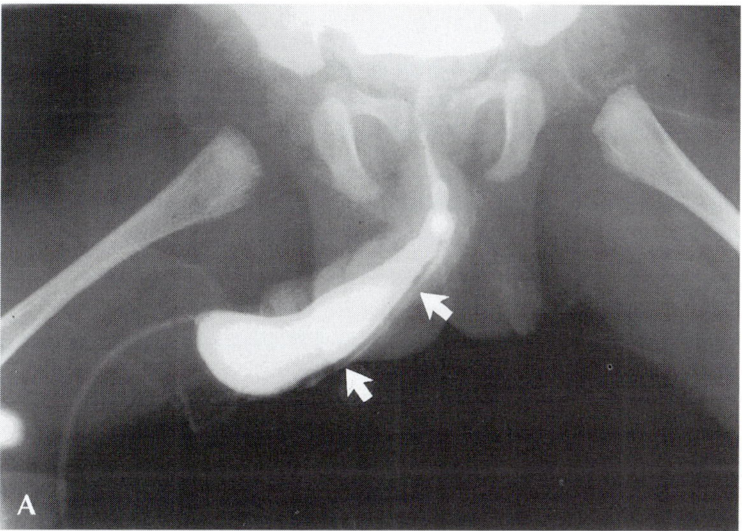

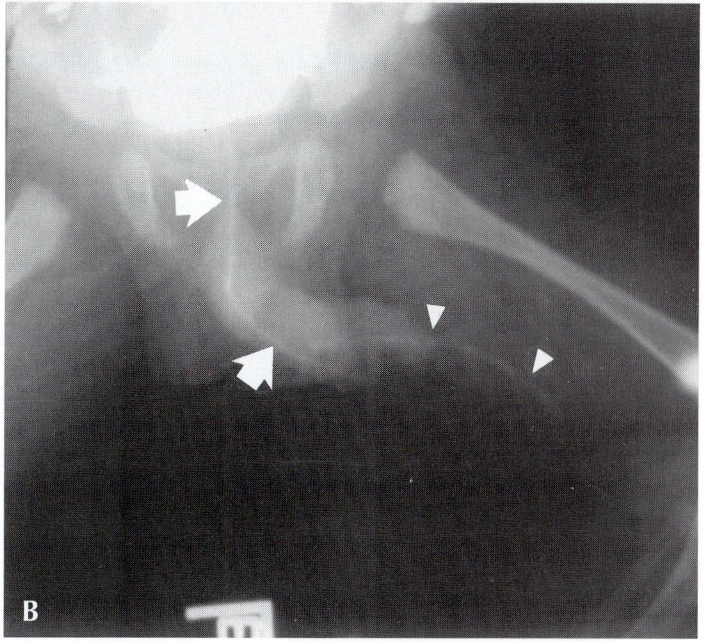

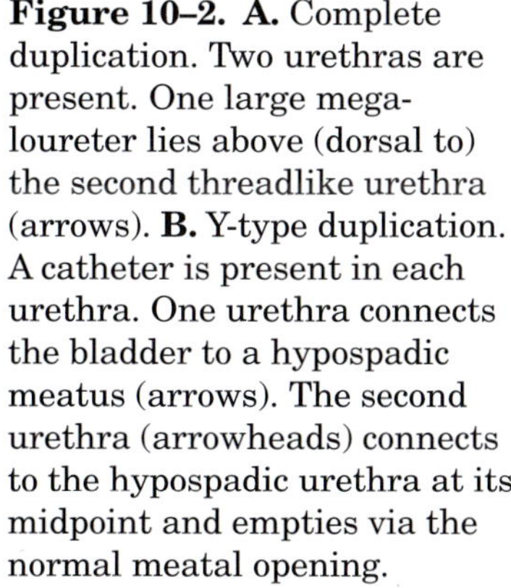
Figure 10–2. A. Complete duplication. Two urethras are present. One large megaloureter lies above (dorsal to) the second threadlike urethra (arrows). **B.** Y-type duplication. A catheter is present in each urethra. One urethra connects the bladder to a hypospadic meatus (arrows). The second urethra (arrowheads) connects to the hypospadic urethra at its midpoint and empties via the normal meatal opening.

have a meatus but instead simply end in periurethral tissues.

Scaphoid Megalourethra

Megalourethra occurs when there is abnormal development of the corpus spongiosum. An abnormality of the corpus cavernosum may also be evident. The penile urethra becomes quite dilated but there is no evidence of obstruction. This abnormality is seen in prune-belly syndrome. It may be seen in other disorders including megaureter and megacystis. There may be associated vesicoureteral reflux.

Anterior Urethral Valve

An anterior urethral valve is a misnomer. The "valve" is a valvelike action that occurs as a result of a urethral diverticulum. The diverticulum occurs ventrally in the penile portion of the anterior urethra. Anterior valves probably occur as the result of anomalous development of the corpus spongiosum or incomplete formation of the urethra. The diverticulum fills with urine when the patient is voiding. Filling of the diverticulum leads to narrowing and obstruction of the urethra (Fig. 10–3). Prominent dribbling is a symptom. Patients may also present with recurring bladder infections. Occasionally, patients develop complete obstruction of the urethra as the diverticulum fills. Retrograde urethrography must be performed to detect this.

Urethral Diverticulum in a Female

Most diverticula of the female urethra probably occur as a result of a periurethral infection of Skene's glands. An alternate

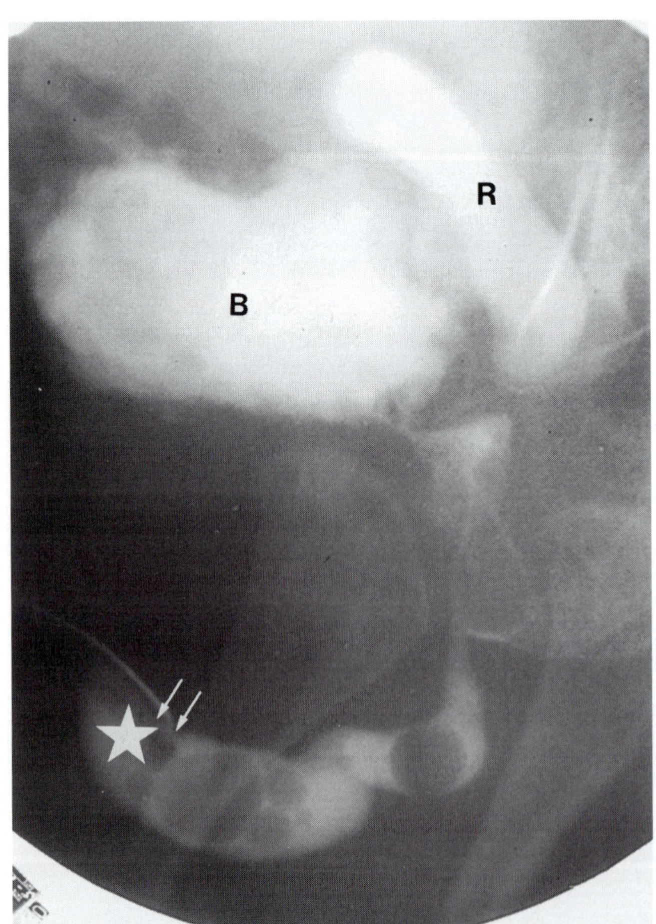

Figure 10–3. A urethrogram with an anterior urethral valve. The catheter enters the meatus. The flap of tissue cannot be seen but is approximately where the small arrows point. This flap causes ballooning of the anterior urethra (star). Air bubbles are visible in the dilated urethra. B = bladder, R = reflux in ureter.

theory postulates that they result from birth trauma. The gland may become obstructed. An abscess forms in the gland and ruptures into the periurethral tissue, resulting in a diverticulum. Patients may present with dribbling, dyspareunia, or, more commonly, recurrent infection. Many of these diverticula will develop stones, and the diverticula that contain stones have an increased risk of adenocarcinoma. The diverticulum may be detected on a postvoid film of intravenous urography or during excretory urography. It may also sometimes be seen in voiding cystourethrography (Fig. 10–4). Radiographically, it may appear as a double density on the voiding film or may retain contrast on a postvoid film and appear as a smooth, round density overlying the region of the urethra. The best demonstration is via retrograde urethrography.

These diverticula occur most commonly in the middle or distal urethra. A small percentage will occur in the proximal urethra. If the urethra projects posteriorly, the diverticulum may extend up in the plane between the urethra and vagina. In this situation, this lesion may produce an indentation on the base of the bladder, which has been referred to as the female prostate.

Posterior Urethral Valves

Posterior urethral valves occur almost exclusively in male infants. The earlier the diagnosis, the greater is the chance that renal function can be preserved. Posterior urethral valves result from abnormal fusion of the plicae colliculi. These are vestigial remnants of the Wolffian duct orifices.

Posterior urethral valves are classified into three types. Type 1 accounts for almost all cases. These extend inferiorly from the distal verumontanum (Fig. 10–5). Type 2 valves are folds of mucosa found near the bladder neck. These are probably not true valves but are due to bladder obstruction. Type 3 valves have a membrane with a central hole. It acts like an iris and is usually at the lower level of the verumontanum.

Diagnosis is made by voiding cys-

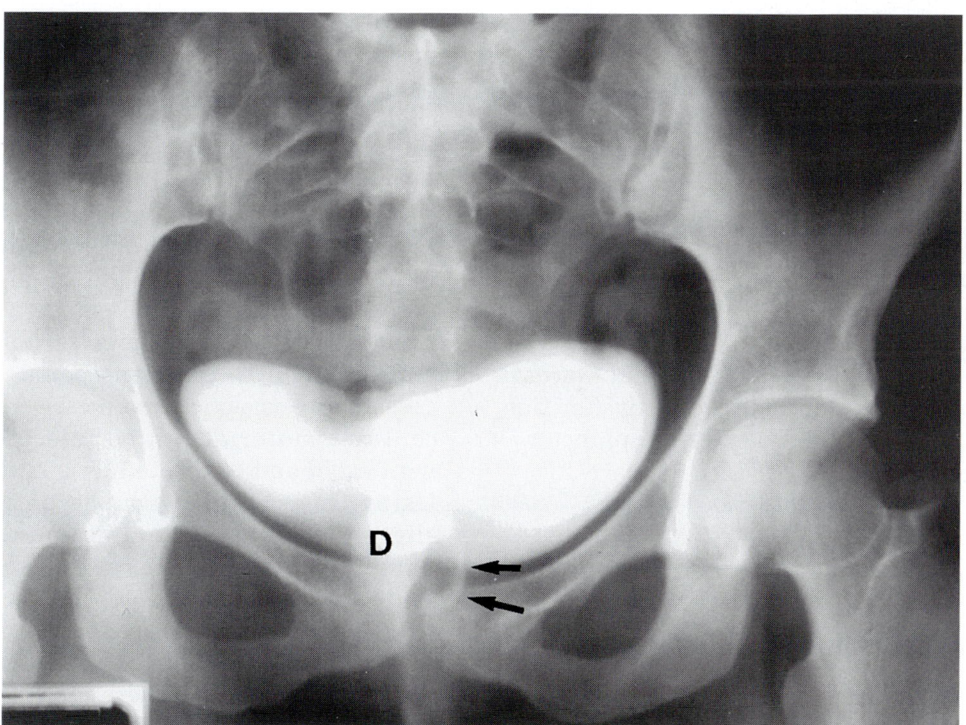

Figure 10–4. An AP film from intravenous urography shows a diverticulum (D) from the posterior urethra. Arrows indicate the urethra.

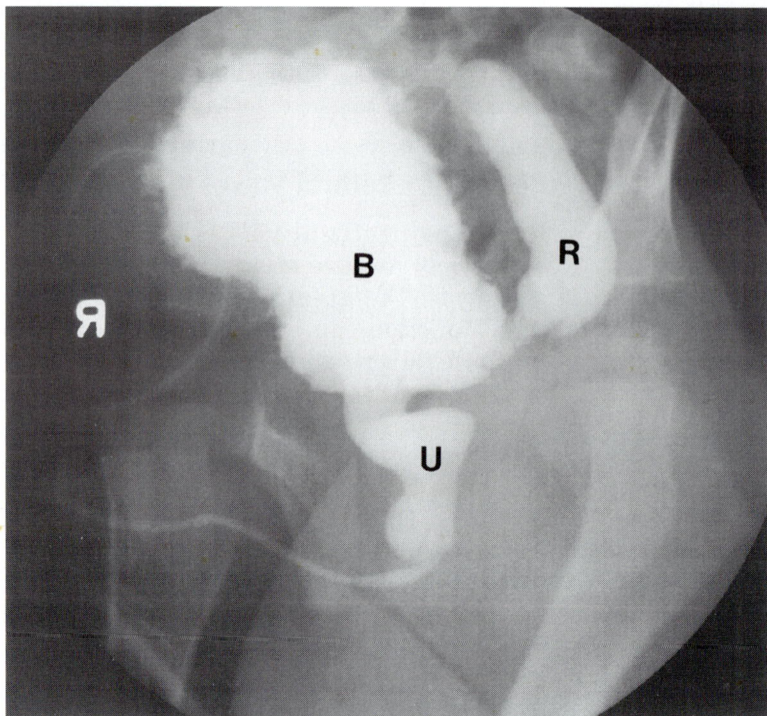

Figure 10–5. Posterior urethral valves. A voiding cystourethrogram showing a dilated posterior urethra (U) and reflux (R) into the left ureter. B = bladder.

tourethrography. Many cases are suspected on the basis of in utero ultrasonographic examinations, in which hydronephrosis, hydroureter, and a distended bladder are seen. At voiding cystourethrography, the bladder wall will usually be thickened and trabeculated, and may show vesicoureteral reflux. Urinary ascites is common. Radiographically, the posterior urethra proximal to the obstructing valve shows a triad of dilatation, elongation, and indentation (of the bladder neck). The bulging valve is often referred to as a "spinnaker sail." Differential diagnosis includes normal mucosal folds, stricture, and neurogenic dysfunction with dyssynergia of the external sphincter.

TRAUMA

Ruptured Corpus Cavernosum

A fracture or rupture of the corpus cavernosum is sometimes referred to as a fracture of the penis. This is most commonly seen as a result of vigorous sexual activity in which the male is on the bottom and the female partner forcibly sits on an erect penis. The patient will complain of severe pain and swelling. The current treatment of choice is operative repair.

A corpora cavernosogram may be used for preoperative planning. The penis is cleansed with Betadine and a small butterfly needle is inserted from the lateral side into one or the other of the corpora cavernosa. This puncture site is made a few centimeters proximal to the external meatus and proximal to the glans penis. The two corpora cavernosa communicate freely, and contrast material can be injected in one with rapid and complete filling of the other. Using fluoroscopy, with the patient in a slightly oblique position, 30 percent iodinated contrast material is injected slowly and multiple views of the penis are obtained. Usually extravasation will be identified at the point of fracture. If no extravasation occurs, there may be an area of the penis that does not enhance. This can be inferred to be the site of the fracture. It may be necessary to do a retrograde examination of the urethra because of associated urethral injuries.

Urethral Trauma

The female urethra is rarely injured except during birth trauma. Traumatic injuries to the male urethra are more common. An injury to the urethra in the region of the prostate and GU diaphragm (prostatomembranous urethra) is associated with pelvic fracture. Approximately 10 percent of patients with a pelvic fracture will have an injury to the urethra. This injury occurs in severe decelerating injuries where the prostatic urethra is sheared off the genitourinary diaphragm. Patients will frequently present with blood in the urethral meatus. Some patients will be unable to void or will have difficulty voiding.

Injuries to the posterior urethra are classified as Type 1, which involves stretching of the urethra but no frank tear; Type 2, which is partial or complete disruption at the prostatomembranous junction (Fig. 10–6); and Type 3, which is a complete disruption near the membranous urethra that extends through the GU diaphragm.

Retrograde urethrograms reveal no extravasation in Type 1 injuries, although the urethra may be elongated and narrower than normal. With Type 2 injuries, extravasation of contrast material will occur but the contrast material will be contained above the GU diaphragm (Fig. 10–6). Type 3 injuries are characterized by extravasation of contrast material on both sides of the GU diaphragm (Fig. 10–7). This contrast material may even reach the base of the bladder and be confused with leaking of contrast material from the bladder. The Type 3 injury is the most common. In general, when suspicion for urethral trauma exists, a catheter should not be passed through the urethra until it is certain that there is no injury to the urethra by a retrograde study. If the patient has already had a catheter passed, a retrograde study can be performed around the catheter.

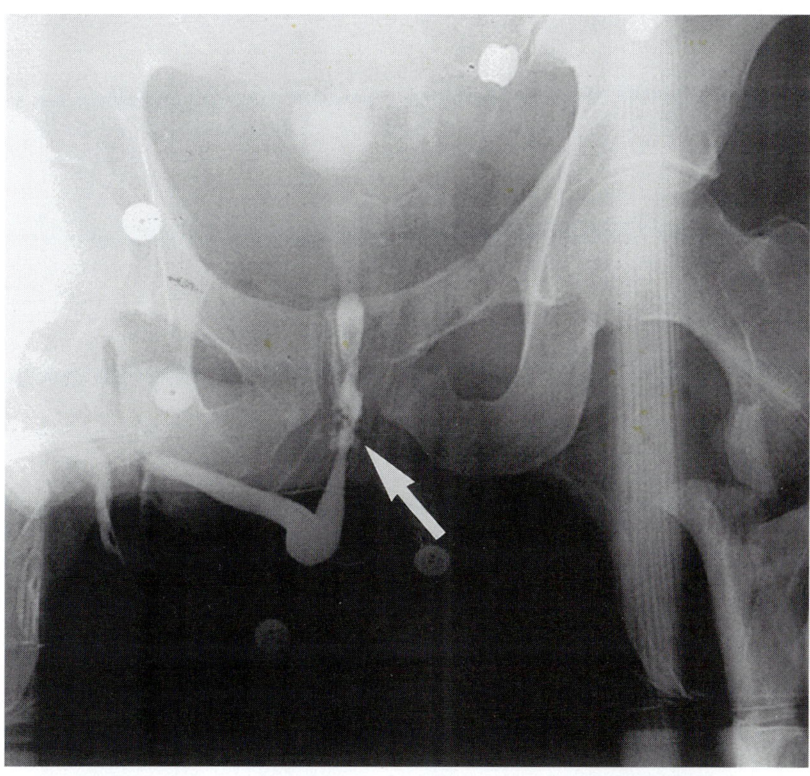

Figure 10–6. A Type 2 urethral injury. There is partial disruption at the prostatomembranous junction with extravasation of contrast material (arrow). The GU diaphragm is intact in this type of injury, and there is no contrast material below this diaphragm.

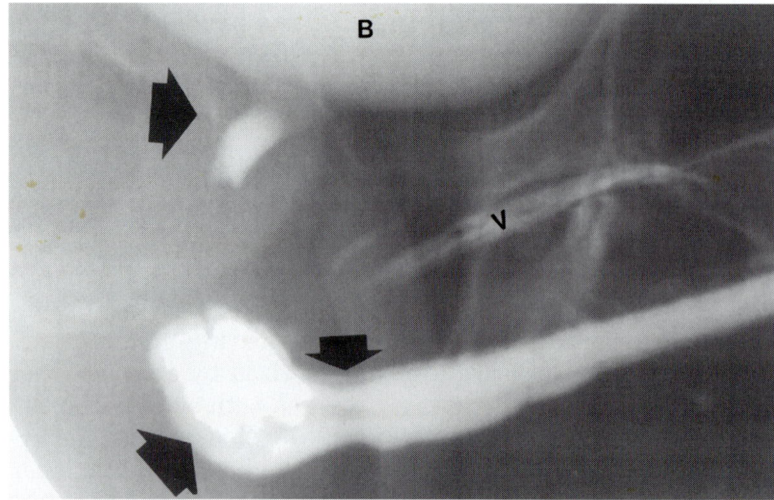

Figure 10–7. A Type 3 injury at presentation. The urethra is completely disrupted, and there was extravasation of contrast material (arrows) both above and below the GU diaphragm, indicating that this diaphragm is disrupted. This is a simultaneous antegrade (through a suprapubic catheter) and retrograde study done days after the injury. V = draining vein, B = bladder.

Urethral Trauma, Anterior Urethra

Injuries of the bulbous urethra may occur as the result of a straddle-type injury in which the patient falls astride a bar, tree limb, or some other cylindrical object and compresses the bulbous urethra against the symphysis. The result may be a localized stricture of the bulbous urethra. In minor injuries the urethra is contused, but intact (Fig. 10–8). Severe injuries may rupture the urethra, with hematoma spreading throughout the perineum and scrotum. Treatment of a minor injury involves placement of a Foley catheter for a few days. If the retrograde urethrogram shows extravasation of con-

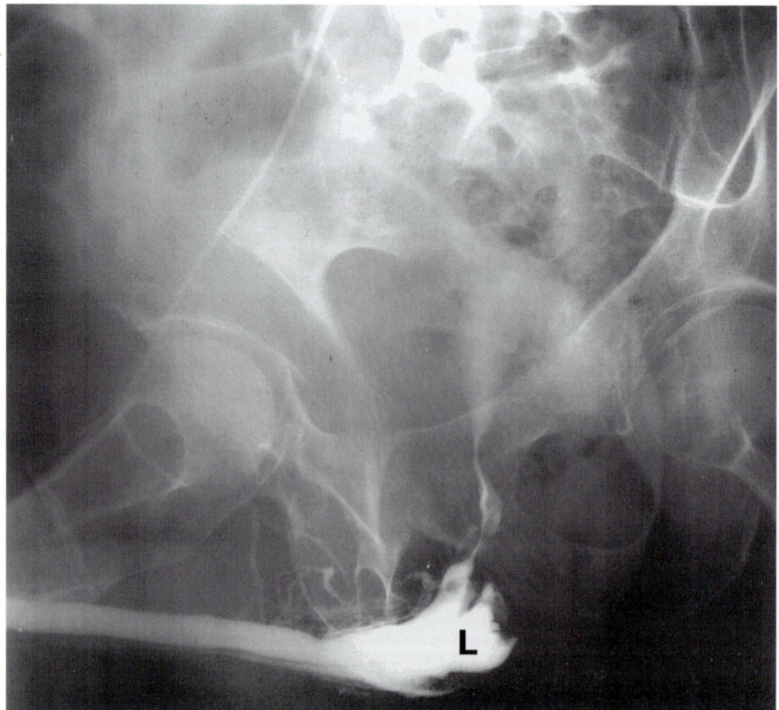

Figure 10–8. A straddle injury with rupture of the bulbous urethra. Contrast material is leaking from the urethra and the filling the draining veins. L = leaking contrast.

trast material, indicating rupture of the urethra, a suprapubic cystostomy is usually performed. If there is extensive extravasation, surgical repair may be necessary. Other anterior urethral injuries include iatrogenic injuries secondary to instrumentation and injuries that are self-induced as a result of intraurethral masturbation.

URETHRITIS AND STRICTURES

Gonorrhea is a common cause of urethritis of the anterior urethra. The glands of Littre become inflamed and scarred, resulting in strictures. On urethrography, these strictures are a few centimeters in length and irregular (Fig. 10–9). The glands of Littre may fill with contrast along the dorsal urethra. Chlamydia is also a common cause of urethritis but is a less common cause of strictures. Rarely, tuberculosis may cause strictures. Fistula formation is common in tuberculosis stricture of the urethra. In the Middle East, *Schistosoma haematobium* is a frequent cause of strictures. A small percentage of patients with condyloma acuminata will get urethral warts or even bladder warts. Strictures may occur for reasons other than infection, including after instrumentation, after a long-term, indwelling catheter, and after pelvic fractures and straddle injuries. Retrograde urethrography will usually show a long, irregular narrowing of the urethra if inflammatory strictures are the cause.

URETHRAL NEOPLASMS

Tumors may produce filling defects on retrograde urethrography. Benign urethral tumors include fibroepithelial polyps in boys. They cause a filling defect in the posterior urethra. Papillomas or adenomatous polyps may have a similar appearance. Malignant tumors usually occur in the bulbous urethra or penile urethra. These are usually squamous cell carcinomas.

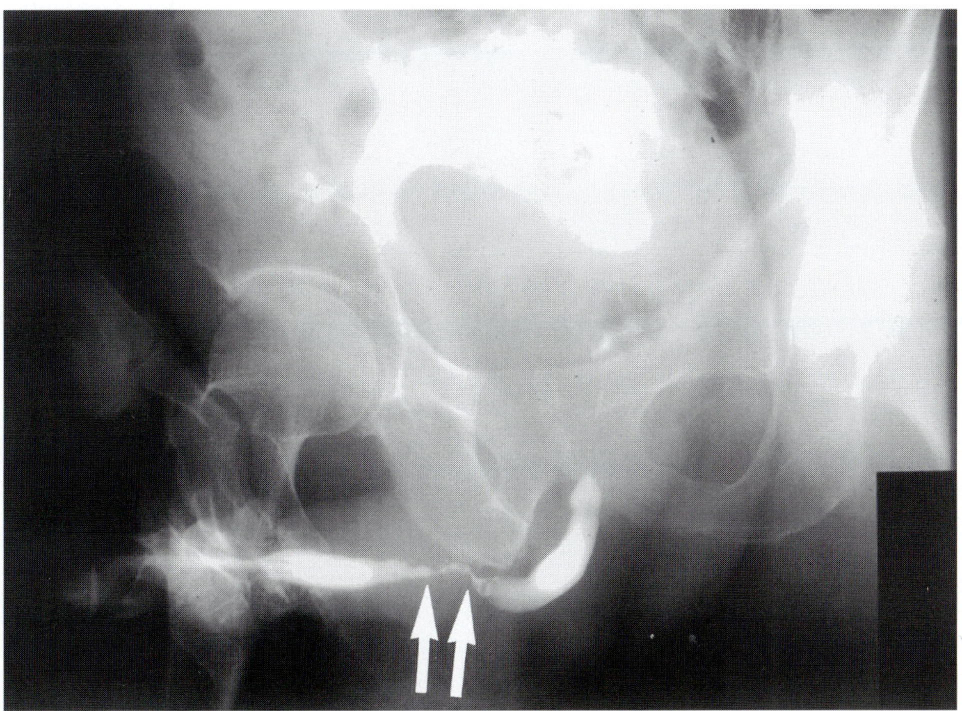

Figure 10–9. An inflammatory stricture (arrows) from gonococci.

Transitional cell carcinomas usually occur as an extension of bladder cancer in the prostatic urethra. Adenocarcinomas occur in the bulbous or membranous urethra, possibly from Cowper's or Littre's glands. Transitional cell carcinoma of bladder and prostate carcinoma are usually sources of primary tumors that extend to the urethra.

PERIURETHRAL CAVITIES

On urethrograms, structures alongside the urethra may occasionally fill, especially if there is a stricture leading to elevated urethral pressures. The glands of Littre are linear, paralleling the dorsal anterior urethra. Cowper's glands may opacify in the genitourinary diaphragm on either side of the urethra, while the ducts may fill in a retrograde fashion in the bulbous urethra.

If pressures are increased in the prostatic urethra, contrast may fill a dilated utricle, which is posterior to the verumontanum. Filling of prostatic ducts may also occur. If the bladder neck is obstructed, reflux into ejaculatory ducts and vas deferens may occur. Extravasation of contrast beneath Buck's fascia of the penis or into veins in the perineum may occur with high-pressure injection and may confuse the interpretation for determination of extravasation.

FEMALE URETHRA

If the female urethra is affected by sexually transmitted diseases, it is usually via pelvic infection instead of as a primary infection.

Tumors of the female urethra present with urinary tract infective symptoms. These occur in the distal two-thirds and are usually squamous cell carcinomas.

Diverticula in females (secondary to infection of Skene's glands) may lead to dyspareunia or symptoms similar to infection. These may be detected with perineal ultrasound or endovaginal ultrasound and may contain stones.

Chapter

11

Testes

NORMAL TESTES

Testes are usually examined by ultrasound, although sometimes MRI, nuclear medicine, and CT are also utilized. Ultrasonography of the normal testes reveals homogeneous egg-shaped structures (Fig. 11–1). Most patients will have a few milliliters of fluid around at least one of the testes. This is a normal finding and should not be considered to be a pathologic hydrocele. The head of the epididymis can be identified in a posterolateral location at the upper pole of the testicle. It will measure 1 cm or less in diameter and will be isodense to the testicle itself. The remainder of the epididymis is harder to identify. The body of the epididymis is a smaller hypoechoic structure extending from the head or caput to the slightly more bulbous tail or caudal epididymis. The tunica vaginalis cannot be discreetly identified by ultrasound or other imaging techniques. There is a bare area around the posterior portion of the testicle where vessels and ducts enter and exit. In addition, the tunica albuginea surrounds and protects the testicle but is not generally visualized either. The tunica albuginea invaginates into the testicle as a structure known as the mediastinum testes.

Sperm traveling from the testicle first travel in the seminiferous tubules. These merge to form the rete testis, which in turn drain into the efferent ductules and epididymis. Capsular arteries supply blood to the testes from the periphery via radiating centripetal arteries. These arteries branch into recurrent rami. Many testes have large arteries that supply the testes via the mediastinum.

Nuclear testicular scans are performed utilizing technetium 99m pertechnetate. This substance is injected by bolus into an arm vein. For the first minute after injection one image is obtained every 4 seconds to check blood flow to the testicle. Several delayed images are obtained after several minutes (Fig. 11–2). Normal testicles show symmetric activity on both flow images and delayed images.

Magnetic resonance imaging of the testicles is usually performed for the evaluation of a tumor. A small surface coil is placed anterior to the testicles. Thin slices are obtained using T1- and T2-weighting parameters (Fig. 11–3). The normal testicles are bright on T2-weighted images.

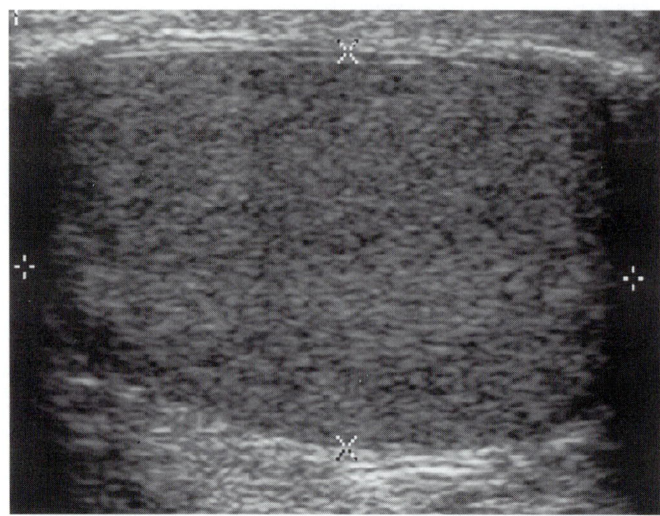

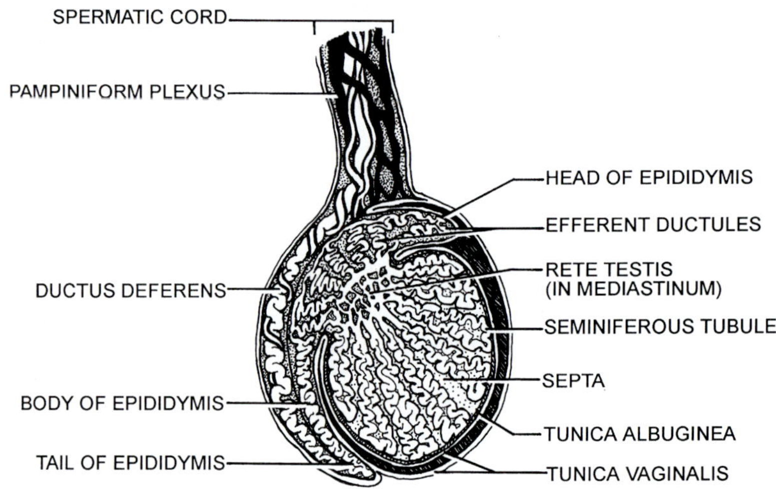

Figure 11–1. A. A normal testicular ultrasound, sagittal image. The testicle should be homogeneous. **B.** A schematic of the testicles. The tunica albuginea is closely applied to the testicles. The tunica vaginalis consists of two layers with potential space in between.

PRIMARY TESTICULAR CANCER

Testicular neoplasms are the most common tumors in males between the ages of 25 and 35, although there is a second peak after age 60. These tumors are classified as either germ cell or stromal tumors (Table 11–1). Almost 90 to 95 percent of testicular tumors are germ cell tumors. Germ cell tumors are classified as either seminomas or nonseminomas. Nonseminomatous tumors include embryonal carcinomas, teratomas, teratocarcinoma, and choriocarcinoma.

Seminomas account for approximately 40 percent of germ cell tumors and are radiosensitive. These are usually hypoechoic at ultrasound and well defined (Fig. 11–4*A*).

Embryonal cell carcinomas are a juvenile variant of yolk sac carcinoma, are radioresistant, and have a greater propensity for early metastatic spread. Necrosis and hemorrhage give this tumor a more disorganized, less well-defined appearance at ultrasound.

Teratomas and teratocarcinomas are part of a spectrum of tumors that contain two or more tissue elements. Teratomas, which occur in prepubescent children and have no identifiable malignant elements at histology, are considered benign. The same tumor in postpubescent males is presumed malignant. Metastases may occur in up to one-third of these patients. Teratocarcinomas have an appearance similar to embryonal cell carcinoma, with inhomogeneity, cystic areas, and frequently calcifications. Choriocarcinoma is seen in adults and

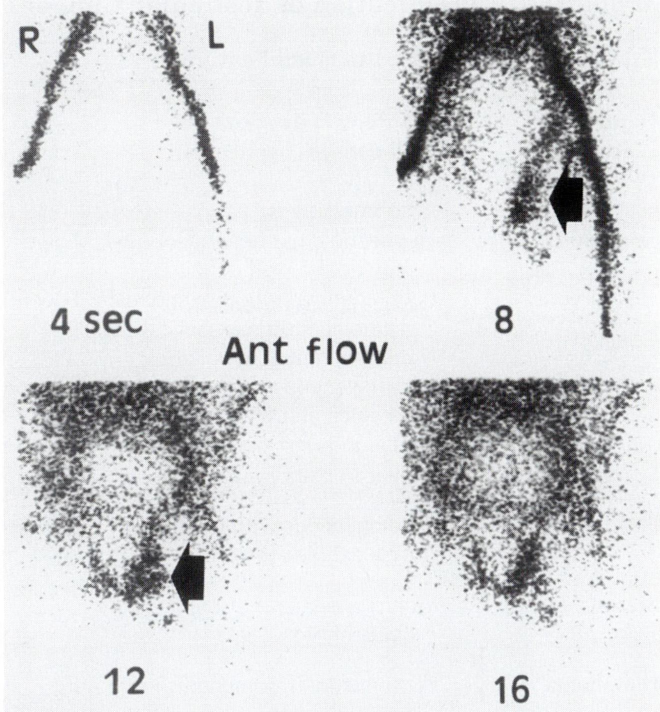

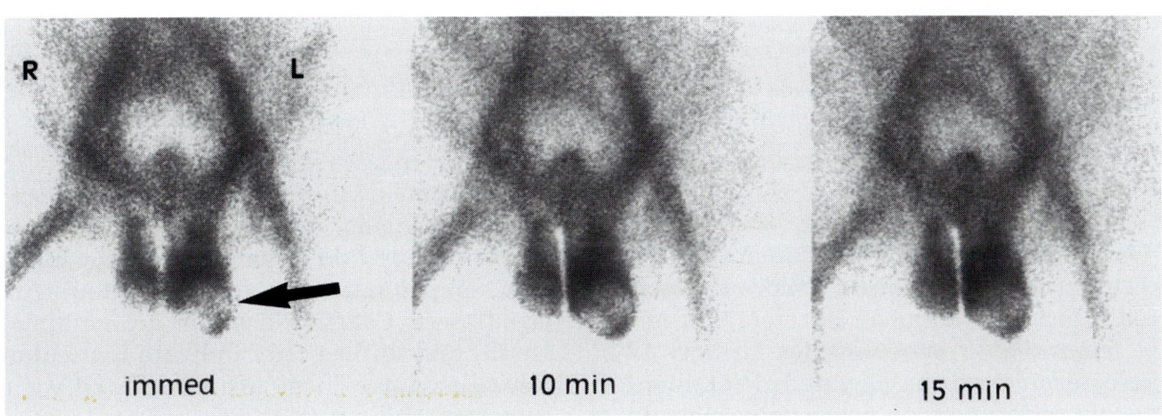

Figure 11–2. **A.** A testicular scan with flow images at 4, 8, 12, and 16 seconds showing increased flow to the left testicle (arrow). **B.** Static images show a focal defect from a testicular abscess (arrow).

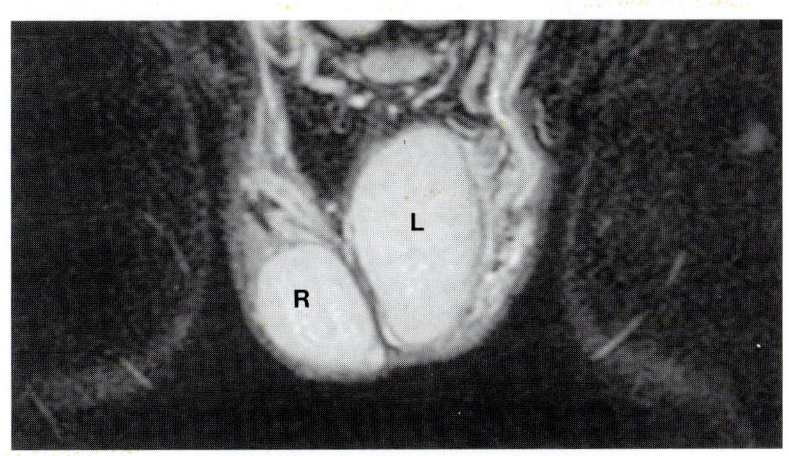

Figure 11–3. A normal MRI of the testicle. This T2-weighted coronal image shows homogeneous high signal in the right (R) and left (L) testicles.

TABLE 11–1. **Classification of Testicular Cancer**

Type	Ultrasound Features	MRI Features	Comments
Germ Cell			
Seminoma	Well-defined, hypoechoic, homogeneous	Lower than testis on T2 images	40% of testicular neoplasms
Mixed	Hypoechoic but heterogeneous, may not be well defined	Lower than testis on T2 images, often heterogeneous	40% of tumors have multiple elements
Embryonal	Poorly defined inhomogeneous, ± calcification may have cysts, predominantly hypoechoic	Low on T2, heterogeneous	20% of tumors
Teratoma	Inhomogeneous, cystic areas, ± calcifications	Low on T2, heterogenous	25% of tumors
Choriocarcinoma	Similar to embryonal	Low on T2	1% of tumors
Yolk sac	Similar to embryonal	Low on T2	
Stromal	Heterogeneous with multiple hypoechoic areas	Low on T2	
Metastases	Multiple, bilateral, usually hypoechoic		GI and GU primaries
Lymphoma	Poorly defined, sometimes infiltrating and difficult to see, usually hypoechoic		Older age group

accounts for only 2 percent of testicular tumors. This is a very aggressive tumor with a poor prognosis.

Stromal tumors are either Leydig cell or Sertoli cell tumors. These tumors tend to occur in 6- to 12-year-old children. Leydig cell tumors are hormone secreters and may be feminizing or masculinizing. Urinary 17-ketosteroids will be elevated. Prepuberal Leydig cell tumors do not usually metastasize, and Sertoli cell tumors are usually benign. At ultrasound these tumors have a heterogeneous appearance with multiple cystic areas throughout the testes. Sertoli cell tumors may have large calcifications with acoustic shadowing. They may be bilateral.

Lymphoma may be of primary testicular origin or may be a result of systemic lymphoma. This tumor makes up one-third of testicular tumors in those over age 50. Lymphomas may be difficult to see on ultrasound but can almost always be seen on MRI. The tumor may be infiltrating, causing a subtle disorganized appearance, or may be a poorly defined hypoechoic mass.

All of these tumors usually have an appearance on T2-weighted MRI scans of a low-signal mass (Fig. 11–4*B*).

Calcifications in the testes may be indicators of malignancy. The isolated focal calcification is usually from a phlebolith, prior infection, or prior trauma and is of doubtful significance. Calcifications that are multiple, small, and diffuse may indicate testicular microlithiasis. These are associated with germ cell tumors (Fig. 11–5). These occur from degenerating cells in seminiferous tubules. These patients should be followed closely. A small cluster of calcifications may be a marker for embryonal cell carcinoma or teratocarcinoma. Other causes of testicular calcifications include sarcoidosis and tuberculosis.

Testicular Cysts

Cysts within the testicle are common, usually seen in older age groups, and frequently near the mediastinum. These are probably a result of dilation of the rete testes. Cysts may be associated with neoplasia, but in this case, the cysts are usually

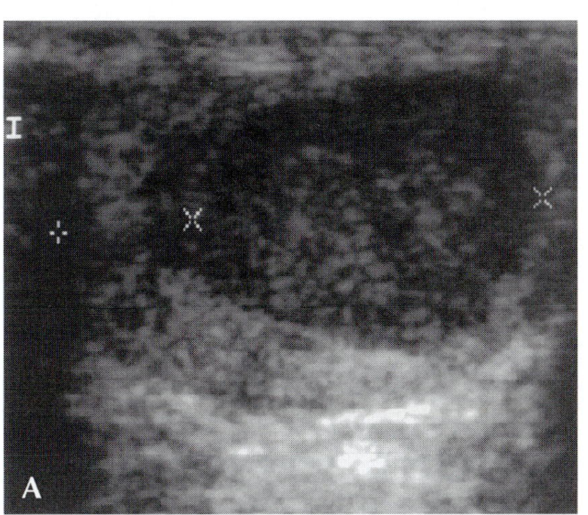

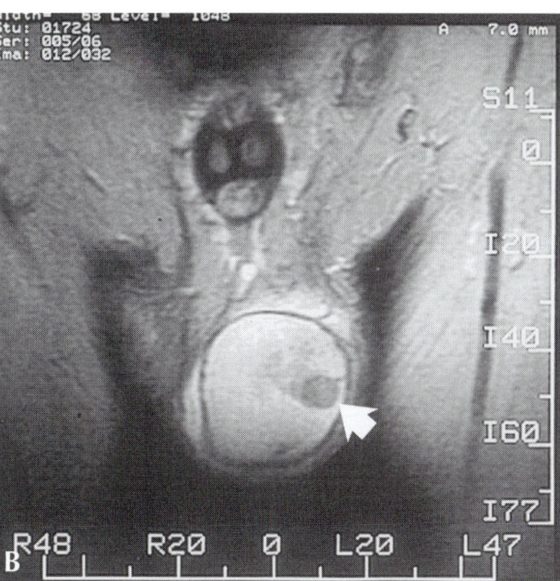

Figure 11–4. **A.** Ultrasound of a testicular tumor. A hypoechoic seminoma is located between the X's. **B.** A coronal image of a T2-weighted MRI of the left testicle shows a low-signal area (arrow) of a seminoma.

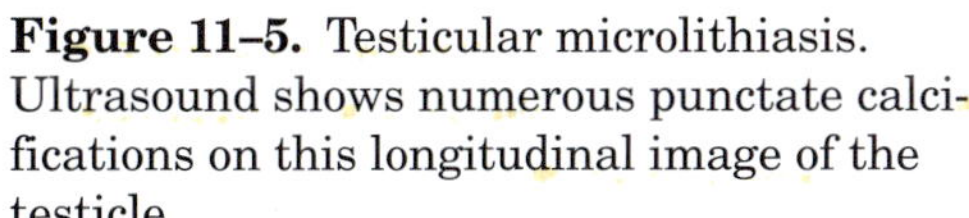

Figure 11–5. Testicular microlithiasis. Ultrasound shows numerous punctate calcifications on this longitudinal image of the testicle.

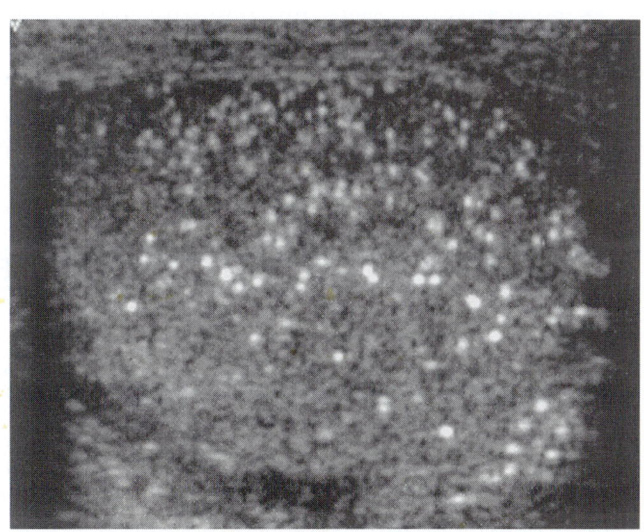

nonsimple with thick walls, irregular contours, and solid components.

EXTRATESTICULAR TUMORS

The most common extratesticular tumor is the adenomatoid tumor. These are usually well defined and homogeneous. They may occur anywhere along the epididymis or even in the spermatic cord, but are usually near the epididymal tail. They are usually a few centimeters in diameter and are a benign tumor.

Epididymal cysts and spermatoceles (Fig. 11–6) differ only in that epididymal cysts contain clear fluid but spermatoceles contain spermatozoa. Both may result from

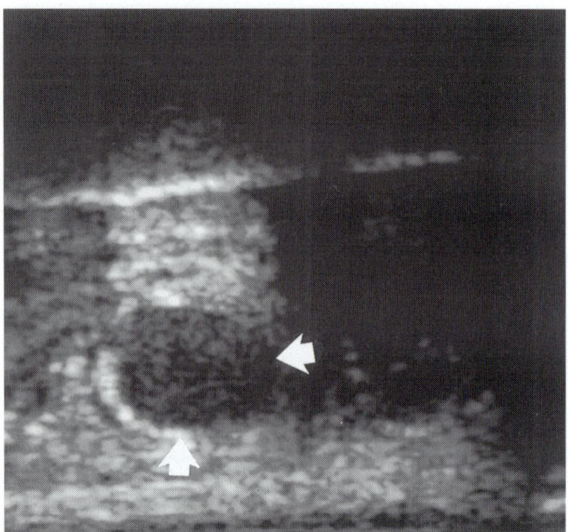

Figure 11–6. Ultrasound of a spermatocele (arrows). Some spermatoceles have low-level echoes such as are seen here.

obstruction of ductules. Both are hypoechoic with good through-transmission and are well circumscribed. They commonly occur near the epididymal head.

Sperm granulomas occur after vasectomy and result from extravasation of sperm with resultant granuloma formation. They are usually solid, hypoechoic, and located near the epididymis.

EPIDIDYMITIS

Epididymitis presents at ultrasound as an enlarged epididymal head. Epididymitis usually results from *Escherichia coli, Pseudomonas* spp., or *Aerobacter* spp. and affects middle-aged men, although any age is susceptible. Clinically, the testicle is painful and tender. Often, fever and a urethral discharge is present. There is usually an associated hydrocele. The hydrocele may have debris or septae in it. The epididymal head is usually larger than 10 mm. Color Doppler imaging of the epididymal head will show increased flow (Fig. 11–7). The remainder of the epididymis (i.e., body and tail) may also be enlarged or thickened. With testicular torsion the epididymal head may be enlarged, so care must be taken to exclude torsion when a large epididymal head is seen.

If epididymitis progresses to orchitis, vague hypoechoic areas may be seen in the testicle. Color Doppler imaging typically often will show increased blood flow.

HYDROCELE

On ultrasound a hydrocele shows hypoechoic fluid in the scrotum in between the visceral and parietal layers of the tunica vaginalis. Almost all males will have at least a small amount of fluid within the scrotum. This small amount of fluid should not be considered to be pathologic. Larger amounts of fluid may occur on an idiopathic basis but should always raise suspicion about possible intrascrotal infection or a tumor. Therefore, whenever a hydrocele is detected, a careful examination of the epididymis and testicle must be performed. Debris or septae within the hydrocele suggest that the fluid may be the result of infection or inflammation.

TESTICULAR TORSION

Torsion of the testicle is a result of a twisting of the testicle with a resultant twisting of the spermatic cord. Arterial blood flow to the testicle becomes obstructed. Testicular torsion has been separated into intravaginal and extravaginal types (Fig. 11–8). The intravaginal type is the more common. As the testicle descends during fetal development, it carries with it a layer of surrounding peritoneum called the tunica vaginalis. In the scrotum this layer will fuse to the underlying tunica albuginea. The posteromedial scrotal wall attaches directly to the testicle because in this area the testicle is not covered by tunica vaginalis. This is known as the bare area. This attached bare area keeps the testicle from rotating within the scrotal sac. This bare area is also a point of entry and exit for vessels. In the

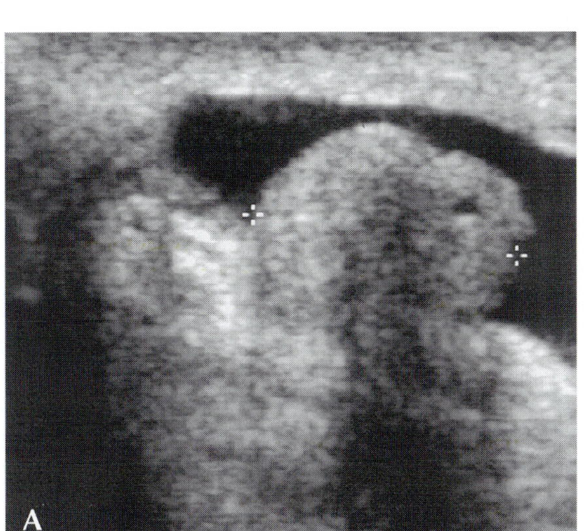

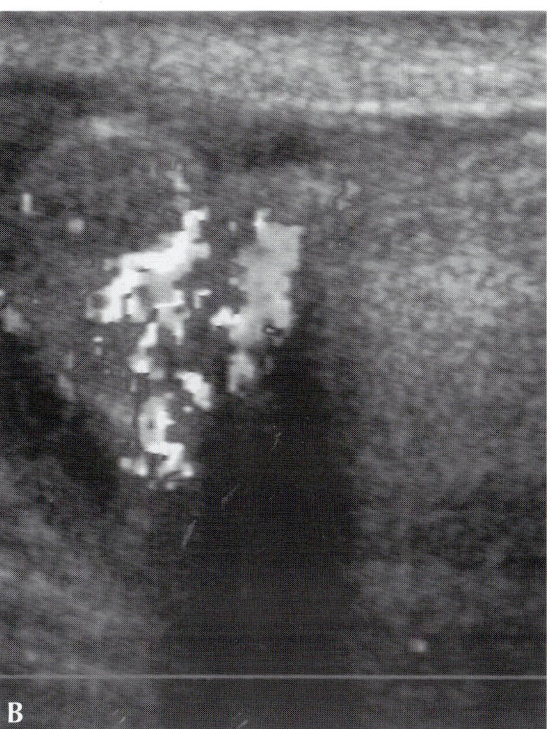

Figure 11–7. Sagittal ultrasound images: **A.** A large epididymal head in a patient with epididymitis. **B.** Color Doppler imaging shows increased flow to the epididymal head.

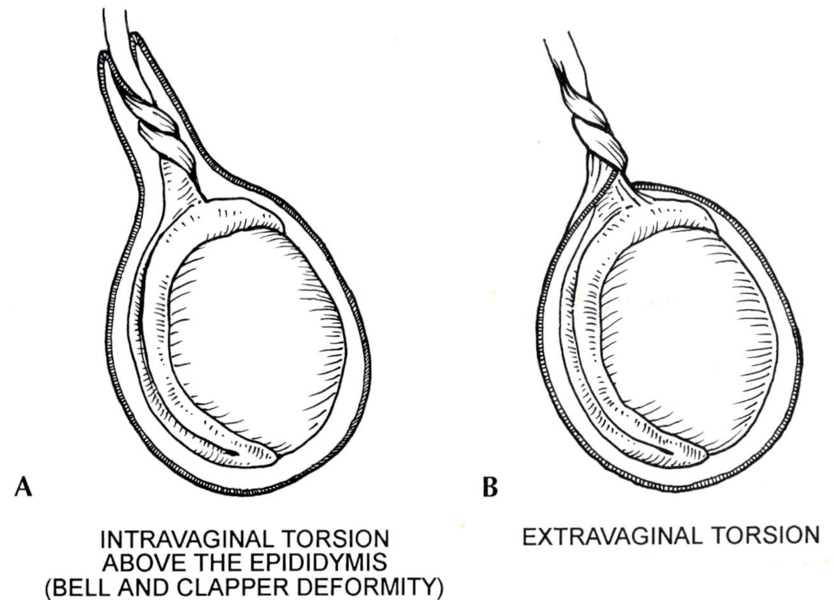

Figure 11–8. A. Intravaginal torsion. The tunica vaginalis inserts high on the cord. The testicle can rotate within the tunica vaginalis and resembles a clapper within a bell. **B.** Normal insertion of the tunica vaginalis. This is called extravaginal torsion.

bell-and-clapper deformity the tunica vaginalis inserts high on the spermatic cord rather than on the scrotum and there is little or no bare area because the tunica vaginalis completely surrounds the testicle. There is a propensity for the testicle to rotate, leading to intravaginal torsion. This condition accounts for the majority of torsed testicles.

Extravaginal torsion results from torsion at the external inguinal ring. This usually occurs perinatally. The tunica attaches normally, but the attachment at the scrotal wall is weak, allowing torsion to occur.

Nuclear scans have been the imaging method of choice to diagnose testicular torsion for a number of years. Technetium-99m pertechnetate is the radioisotope that is used. Dynamic images of arterial blood flow are obtained every 2 seconds for approximately the first minute and then images are obtained every 5 minutes for a total of 20 minutes of imaging. In the first 24 hours after torsion, the testicle will show normal or slightly decreased activity on the flow images obtained from the first minute. The delayed images will show a cold area corresponding to the testicle. As torsion proceeds beyond 24 hours, a testicle will remain cold but collateral blood flow around the scrotum will occur with resultant increased activity. The appearance is that of a hot rim with a central cold area. The appearance is not pathognomonic, as abscess and hematoma may also have a hot rim, reflecting increased flow, with a cold center, reflecting decreased flow. The accuracy of nuclear medicine imaging is felt to be higher than 95 percent.

Color flow Doppler imaging has been used for approximately the past 5 years. It is felt to have an accuracy approaching that of nuclear medicine. With ultrasound, in the first 4 hours, the testicle will have either a normal appearance or may be hypoechoic, reflecting edema. At Doppler ultrasound there will be decreased or no flow. This examination must be done in a meticulous fashion because the flow within the testicle is normally very slow and Doppler techniques to detect slow flow must be used. After the first 24 hours the testicle that has been torsed will have a very heterogeneous echo appearance. Patients who torse and detorse may have a Doppler study that shows normal or even increased flow. That phenomenon can cause problems with color Doppler imaging in the diagnosis of testicular torsion.

Torsion of Appendixes

Torsion of the appendix testis or appendix epididymis can mimic testicular torsion clinically (Fig. 11–9). The former conditions do not need surgical attention. The appendix testis is a vestige of the Müllerian duct remnant. It may torse, usually in preadoles-

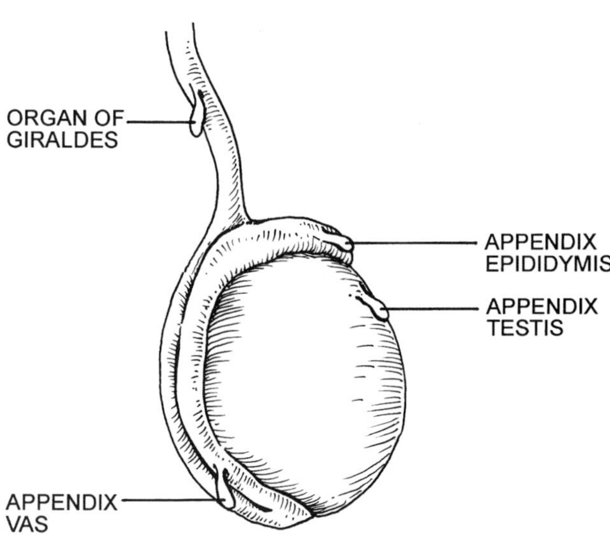

Figure 11–9. A drawing of the four testicular appendixes.

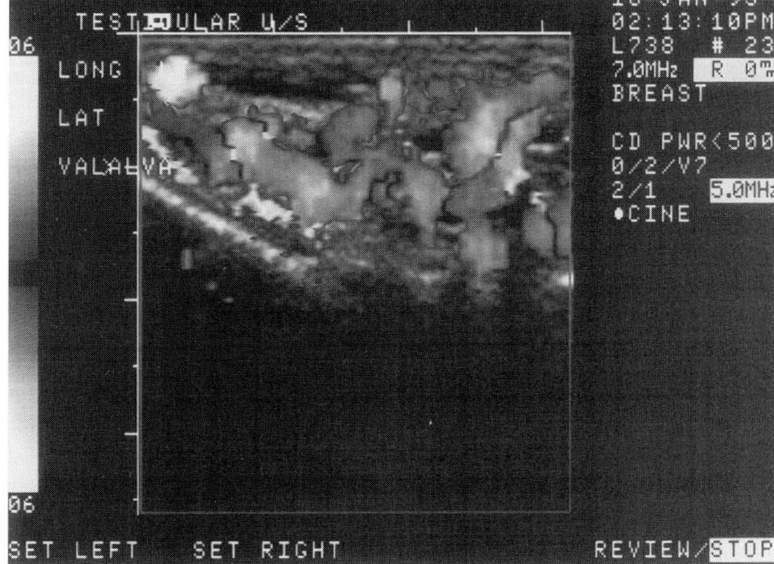

Figure 11–10. A color Doppler image (depicted in black and white) showing dilated veins in the pampiniform plexus of the spermatic cord.

cents, causing pain. These appendixes may sometimes be seen with ultrasound and appear as a small hyper- or hypoechoic mass in an extratesticular location. No treatment is needed for these conditions.

Cryptorchidism

The testes descend into the scrotum at about 36 weeks' gestation, guided by the gubernaculum testes, a structure extending from testis to the inferior scrotum. The incidence is increased dramatically in low-birth-weight and premature infants, although many undescended testes will descend spontaneously before 1 year of age. Nondescended testes may be located anywhere in the retroperitoneum between kidneys and scrotum, although most are in the inguinal canal. Localization of these testes is necessary to prevent infertility and cancer. Descent may then be accomplished surgically.

Ultrasound is usually utilized to find the testes. An egg-shaped structure in the inguinal area is usually found. Magnetic resonance imaging has also been utilized and is especially useful if ultrasound is unsuccessful. If ultrasound and MRI are unsuccessful, CT may be tried. Finally, venography is a highly accurate test, but it is invasive. A catheter is inserted into the femoral vein. The tip of the catheter is advanced until the testicular vein is selected. A retrograde injection is performed, and the venous plexus around the testicle can be reliably identified.

Trauma

After trauma to the testicle, ultrasound may be used to identify rupture prior to surgical intervention. Focal areas of increased or decreased echogenicity may be seen, with fracture planes occasionally identified. Hematoceles may also be seen.

Varicocele

Ultrasound is used to diagnose varicoceles. These can be important in infertility because they warm the testicle, which leads to a decreased sperm count. A vein greater than 2 mm in diameter (Fig. 11–10) should be considered to be a varicocele. Color and pulsed Doppler are used to confirm that the structures being imaged are veins.

Chapter

12

Adrenal Gland

NORMAL ADRENAL GLAND

The normal adrenal gland has a shape that may resemble either an upside down Y or an upside down V (Fig. 12–1). The right adrenal gland is located superior and medial to the kidney. The left adrenal gland is slightly medial to the upper pole of the left kidney. These glands have a variable appearance. In general, a limb of the adrenal gland should not be thicker than 10 mm. Adrenal glands are usually not convex in shape. The adrenal glands are normally scanned with 3-mm cuts at CT. Magnetic resonance imaging of the adrenal is sometimes utilized, but a CT would be the test of choice in most situations.

ADRENAL MASSES

Evaluation of the adrenal gland by plain film is usually unrewarding. Occasionally, adrenocortical carcinoma will have calcifications. Other entities such as adrenal hemorrhage can also calcify, making this finding nonspecific. Intravenous urography will not be helpful unless the adrenal gland is significantly enlarged. There may be an impression on the upper pole of the kidney, or the upper pole may be slightly displaced laterally. Computed tomography is the imaging method of choice for the adrenal gland. An adrenal cyst can readily be identified by the water density within the adrenal lesion. Likewise, fat can be identified on the basis of its CT or Hounsfield number. Fat found in an adrenal lesion is essentially pathognomonic of a myelolipoma or benign adenoma.

Small nodular masses in a limb of the adrenal gland are a common finding on a CT done for other reasons. These are usually adrenal adenomas, and usually they are not hyperfunctioning. As many as 3 percent of people will have an adrenal adenoma. These adenomas can sometimes grow to a huge size and may occasionally calcify. They are usually well defined and homogeneous. At one point it was thought that MRI might be useful to distinguish between an incidental adrenal adenoma and metastatic disease to the adrenal gland. In theory, metastases should have a higher intensity on a T2-weighted sequence. However, this method has not been sufficiently reliable.

Currently, work is being done with the

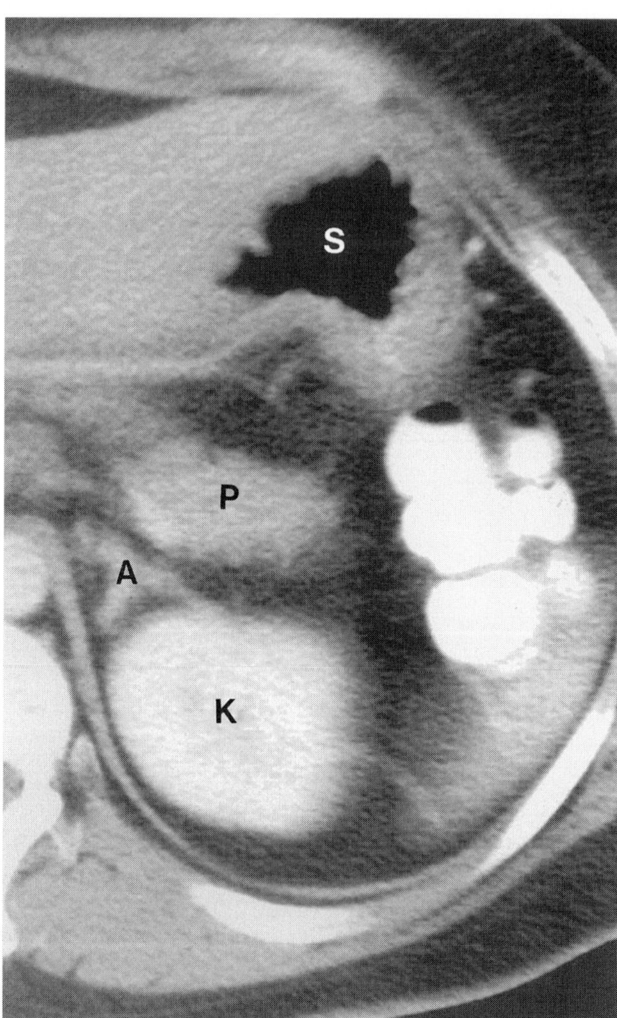

Figure 12–1. An axial CT image coned to the left abdomen showing a normal adrenal gland (A), pancreas (P), and left kidney (K), and stomach gas (S).

use of "in-phase" and "out-of-phase" chemical shift MRI to distinguish between adenomas and metastatic disease to the adrenal glands. In this procedure the adrenal glands are scanned twice. On one scan the image is acquired with an out-of-phase TE, about 2.3 ms at 1.5 tesla. The adrenal gland then is scanned once again with in-phase TE, which is about 4.6 ms. The "out-of-phase" connotation refers to the fact that, at 2.3 ms, fat protons are out of phase with water protons and their signal will cancel out. At 4.6 ms fat protons are in phase with water protons and their signal will be additive. Therefore, a loss of signal in the out-of-phase image (2.3 ms) compared to the in-phase image implies the presence of fat (Fig. 12–2). Fat in an adrenal mass is nearly pathognomonic of an adenoma.

Similar work has been done using CT and its cutoff threshold of 10 H. If noncontrast CT measurements are below 10 H, the sensitivity is 79 percent and the specificity is 96 percent for an adenoma. This method relies on the fact that fat normally measures approximately –60 H and soft tissue will measure +50 or +60 H. The detection of Hounsfield units below +10 suggests the presence of fat and therefore the presence of an adenoma (Fig. 12–3).

Others have used size as a criterion. Since 78 percent of adrenal masses less than 3 cm in diameter are benign adenomas and 91 percent of those greater than 3 cm in diameter are malignant, adrenal masses greater than 6 cm in diameter are almost all malignant and should be removed.

Evaluation of the adrenal glands is pre-

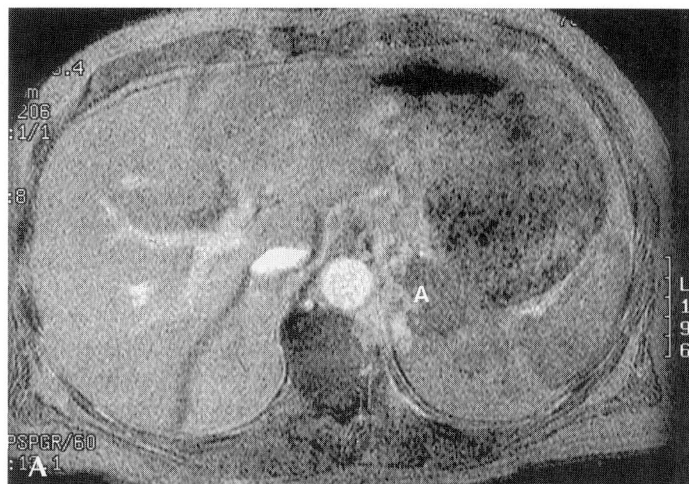

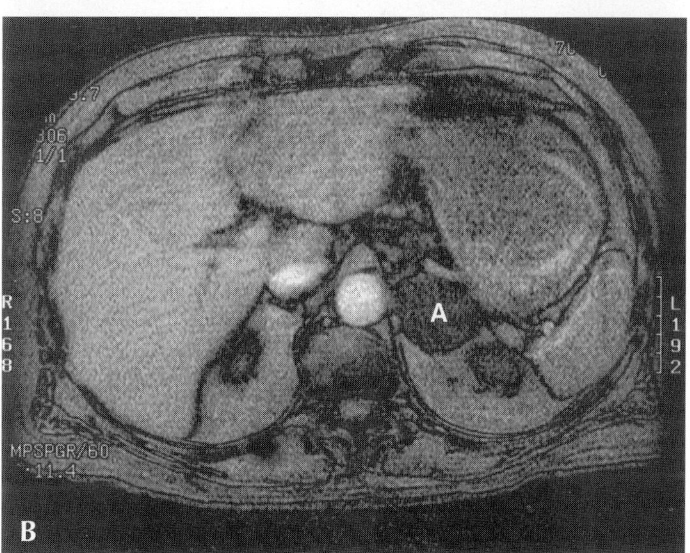

Figure 12–2. In-phase axial MRI **(A)** and out-of-phase axial MRI **(B)** of the left adrenal gland showing signal dropout on out-of-phase images. This decrease in signal intensity indicates the presence of fat, and this allows a diagnosis of adenoma to be made.

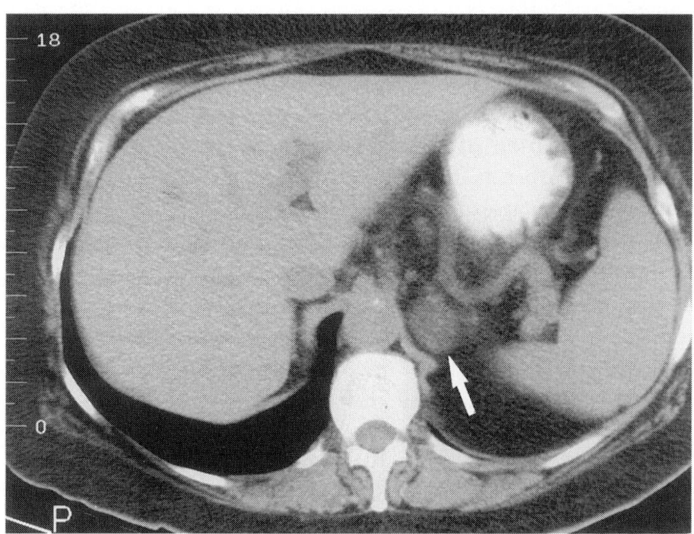

Figure 12–3. Axial CT showing a left adrenal mass (arrow). This mass appears lower in density than adjacent organs and measured –11 H. This indicates fat and allows a diagnosis of adrenal adenoma.

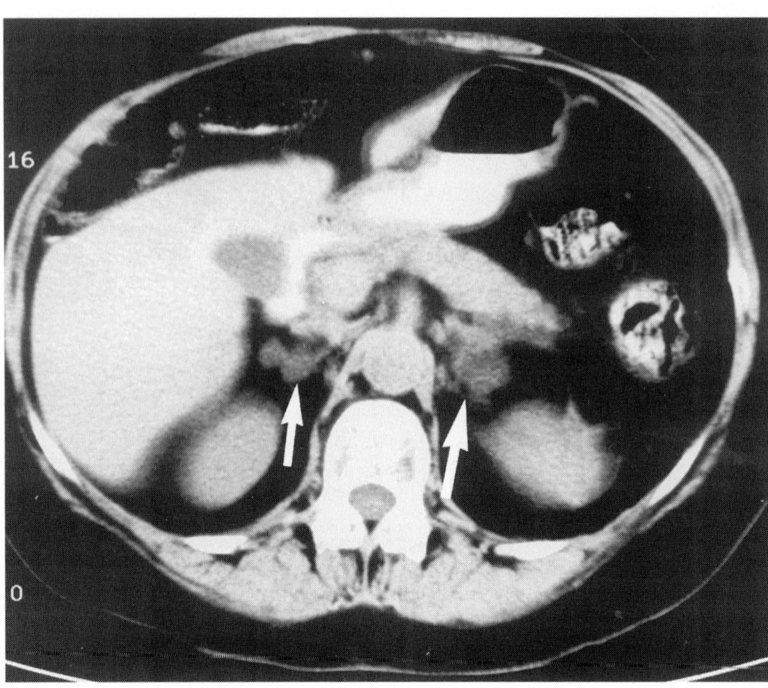

Figure 12–4. Macronodular adrenal hyperplasia. Both adrenal glands have multiple nodules.

cipitated when a clinical diagnosis of Cushing's syndrome occurs. Elevated cortisol results in a "buffalo hump," "moon face," truncal obesity, and excessive fat deposition. About 80 percent of these cases are due to a pituitary adenoma leading to bilateral adrenal hyperplasia, 15 percent are due to an adrenal adenoma, and 5 percent are due to adrenal carcinoma. A small percentage (5 to 10 percent) of cases of adrenal hyperplasia result from ectopic ACTH production by tumors such as oat cell carcinoma tumors, carcinoid, and pheochromocytoma. CT in these patients will sometimes show bilateral diffuse enlargement, although significant numbers (50 percent) will have either normal glands or glands with multiple small nodules (Fig. 12–4). The differentiation of an adenomatous gland from a multinodular gland in hyperplasia, especially if there is a dominant nodule, is challenging. However, this is an important distinction because surgical removal of an adenoma is curative whereas surgical adrenalectomy in hyperplasia is futile because the other gland remains in place. In summary, bilateral increased size or bilateral small nodules suggest hyperplasia, but a prominent nodule with otherwise normal adrenal glands suggests an adenoma.

Primary hyperaldosteronism results from elevated aldosterone levels with resultant hypertension and hypokalemia. Renin levels are suppressed. Eighty percent of these cases have a solitary adrenal adenoma. The other 20 percent have hyperplastic adrenal glands, often with nodules. It may not be possible using CT or MRI to distinguish nodular hyperplastic glands from those with adenomas. In this situation venous sampling for aldosterone levels from adrenal and renal veins is necessary.

A suprarenal mass in a child raises the possibility of neuroblastoma. About one-third of neuroblastomas are in the adrenal gland. These usually occur in the first two years of life. In children, sonography is very useful because of the small amount of body fat. A heterogeneous-appearing mass is identified in the region of the adrenal gland. The differential diagnosis often involves distinguishing neuroblastomas from a Wilm's tumor. This distinction is often made on clinical grounds. Unlike Wilm's tumor, neuroblastoma classically displaces the superior pole of the kidney laterally and inferiorly on intravenous urography. Neuroblastoma also can display stippled calcification on intravenous urography or CT. The distinction between these two tumors has been facilitated with the development of CT imaging.

Adrenal cortical carcinomas may occur in either adrenal gland or may be bilateral. They are more common on the left. They are usually quite large and frequently have a heterogeneous density with evidence of necrosis in the center (Fig. 12–5). Calcification is common. Calcification can be seen more easily on CT than on a plain film. These tumors also commonly invade the inferior vena cava.

Finally, adrenal hemorrhage may cause a large suprarenal mass. This is more common in children but can occur at any age. It usually does not cause adrenal insufficiency. Adrenal hemorrhage can be associated with septicemia, hypertension, or renal vein thrombosis, or it may occur with preexisting adrenal tumors. Anticoagulated patients are at risk. The right adrenal gland hemorrhages more often than the left. If the hemorrhage is relatively acute, the resultant mass will have a high density, with Hounsfield units approaching 100. Over time, the hematoma will start to resolve and the mass will become closer to water density or 0 H.

In summary, the features on CT of a benign adenoma are of a sharply marginated, smooth contoured mass less than 3 cm in size. On the other hand, lesions larger than 6 cm with low-density areas suggestive of necrosis, with calcifications, or with evidence of metastatic spread are suggestive of adrenal cortical carcinoma.

PHEOCHROMOCYTOMA

Pheochromocytomas are usually found in the adrenal gland. Approximately 10 percent may be found in extra-adrenal locations, commonly along the sympathetic chain. They may also be associated with multiple endocrine neoplasia (MEN). Type 2A includes medullary carcinoma of the thyroid, parathyroid hyperplasia, and pheochromocytoma. Type 2B includes medullary carcinoma of the thyroid, pheochromocytoma, and multiple neuromas. Pheochromocytomas are also associated with neurofibromatosis and the von Hippel-Lindau syndrome. Sporadic pheochromocytomas, not

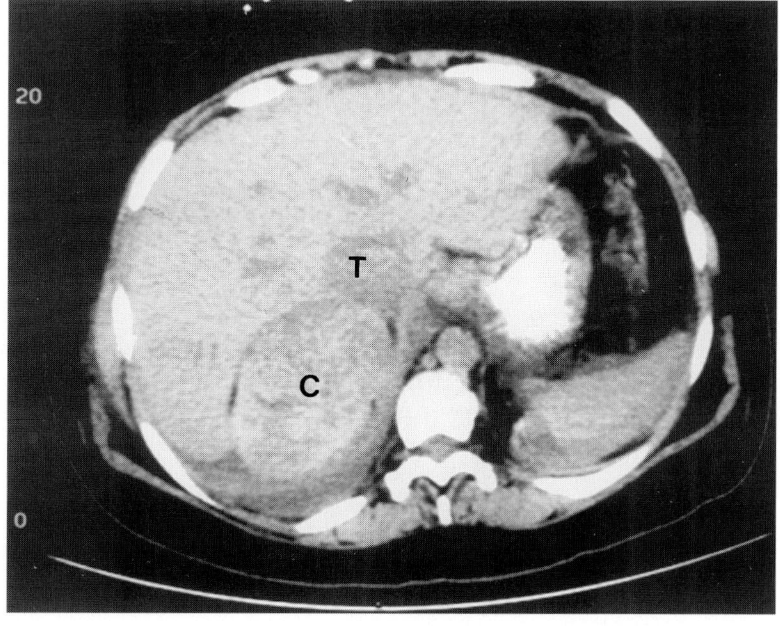

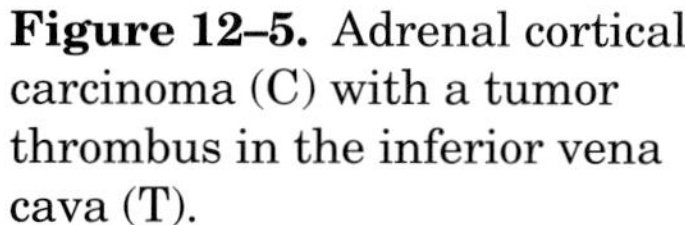
Figure 12–5. Adrenal cortical carcinoma (C) with a tumor thrombus in the inferior vena cava (T).

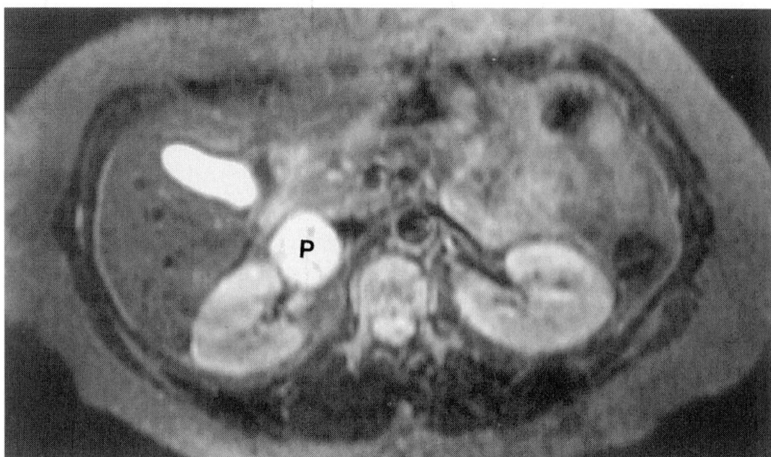

Figure 12–6. Pheochromocytoma. This T2-weighted axial image shows the high signal intensity of an extra-adrenal pheochromocytoma (P).

associated with any of these syndromes, are more likely to be outside of the adrenal gland. Those involved in the MEN 2 syndrome are more often multicentric. Approximately 10 percent of pheochromocytomas will be malignant. The diagnosis is made using a combination of laboratory tests for serum catecholamines and their metabolites, as well as radiographic imaging.

When a patient is scanned using either CT or MRI in an effort to locate a pheochromocytoma, scanning should be performed from at least the diaphragm through the dome of the bladder. If a pheochromocytoma is still not identified and there is a high index of suspicion, it may be worthwhile to expand the scope of imaging to include the base of the skull, chest, and heart. A nuclear medicine test using iodine-labeled metaiodobenzylguanimine (MIBG) has been said to have an accuracy and sensitivity of about 90 percent. The CT appearance of a pheochromocytoma is that of a rounded, well-circumscribed mass measuring several centimeters in diameter. The density ranges from homogeneous to tumors with a low-density center. The low-density center may be due to some necrosis. These tumors occasionally calcify. On MRI these tumors are extremely bright on a T2-weighted image (Fig. 12–6). This finding makes them very conspicuous. MRI has been advocated as a way to screen for pheochromocytomas in patients who have a high index of suspicion.

Index

Note: Page numbers in *italics* indicate illustrations; those followed by t refer to tables.